A Deeper Perspective on Alzheimer's and Other Dementias

Practical Tools with Spiritual Insights

Megan Carnarius, RN, NHA, LMT

FINDHORN PRESS

ISBN: 978-1-84409-662-6

With special thanks to Ken Cohen for the permission to quote from his book
Honoring the Medicine: The Essential Guide to Native American Healing
(Ballantine Books, 2003) in Chapter 15 (The Medicine Wheel) of this book.

Artwork by Megan Carnarius
Artwork digitized by Emily Snyder
Photographs by Liza Weems

Edited by Nicky Leach
Cover design by Richard Crookes
Interior design by Joan Pinkert
Printed and bound in the EU

Published by
Findhorn Press
117–121 High Street
Forres IV36 1AB,
Scotland, UK

t+44 (0) 1309 690582
f+44 (0) 131 777 2711

e info@findhornpress.com
www.findhornpress.com

DISCLAIMER

The information in this book is given in good faith and is
neither intended to diagnose any physical or mental condition
nor to serve as a substitute for informed medical advice or care.
Please contact your health professional for medical advice and
treatment. Neither author nor publisher can be held liable by
any person for any loss or damage whatsoever which may arise
from the use of this book or any of the information therein.

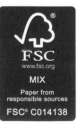

FSC
www.fsc.org
MIX
Paper from
responsible sources
FSC® C014138

....

Contents

Preface

This year is my 25th anniversary of providing care for, and working specifically with, individuals diagnosed with some type of dementia. Over many years of designing programs and facilities and managing these environments, I have worked with hundreds of families, professional caregivers, and individuals with this challenge, and many of those attending my lectures and trainings started requesting that I write a book.

I view myself as someone who is a roll-your-sleeves-up kind of person, so writing a book has been a challenge. To get it to the finish line, it's taken me 14 years, using snippets of time outside of work, while continuing to learn and have the usual ups and downs that life tends to provide. My hope is that this book will be useful to family caregivers as well as professionals in this field, and that individuals in the early stages of a dementia diagnosis will find it helpful as well.

This book is about understanding some of the deeper lessons we are exposed to through caring for individuals with Alzheimer's disease and other dementias. We all want a cure. But in the meantime, while this illness is still with us, how can we create a quality of life for each person in each stage of the disease? How can we look deeper into situations that at first glance look hopeless and destructive in order to find opportunities for insight, inspiration, and greater understanding of ourselves and those we love? How can we allow the full measure of the experience to unfold and be felt with as much of ourselves as we can bring to bear?

Soul-searing, life-testing situations have what some call "fallout blessings." For example, we don't want emergencies, but we certainly are glad that someone knows what to do when we do have them. Without emergencies, a paramedic or emergency nurse would not be able to experience his or her developing skills and abilities to be of service to others. Some prior crisis helped them in navigating the current moment, redirecting it to stable ground.

These silver linings, unexpected graces, or "Yods" as they are known in the Hebrew tradition, can sometimes take a long time to reveal themselves, or a long time to germinate in us. They can also manifest synergistically, becoming quickly visible and profoundly understood. Whether it's a complicated emergence or a seemingly orchestrated lightning bolt, these blessings are often life-affirming and have an objective, substantive impact. They change our lives.

My wish for those who care for those of us going through the difficult dementia journey is that we strive, through the tumultuous waves, to remain awake and open to the blessings of that journey. We are in a vocation in which the gifts brought to us by others can be fully appreciated and recognized, so that this soul-searing experience offers a growth/initiatory process that opens our hearts, nurtures our compassion, and ultimately enables us to be better human beings.

My wish for those brave individuals living with memory loss illnesses is that they be supported and allowed to live their experience fully in their own unique way, to recapitulate, to express, to love and be loved, and to be sheltered from harm. In later stages, they are no longer involved in mundane worldly existence and are in a deep, internal state that we as caregivers generally cannot reach into and share. Dementia has built a wall around them, as if they have entered a cloister. Rather than think of this wall as an imprisonment, I view it as a final honoring of the life this individual has led and of the body or vessel that housed them. Allowed to cocoon, it affords the time needed for the soul to attend to deeper aspects of the self on a spiritual level.

My last hope is that in the final stages, when ready, the individual can let go and be allowed to let go, when they know it's time.

Chapter 1

The Foundation and Vision of Memory Care

Dementia is defined as "severely impaired memory and reasoning ability, usually with disturbed behavior associated with damaged brain tissue." Just as a bone can be malformed at birth, or injured through life experience, the brain also can be malformed initially or injured or altered along the way, making abilities or disabilities occur.

The disease has been part of human experience for a very long time. It undoubtedly occurred prior to recordkeeping, but there are recorded incidences of it in Egyptian and Greek writings.

Cultures have responded in various ways to brain anomalies, and there is a definite correlation between a culture's established, stabilized functioning and its ability to accept and allow demented individuals to coexist in the community. In cases where the survival of the group depended on how productive the individual was and how crucial their contributions were, as in nomadic tribes, they did not have the luxury of sustaining a noncontributor.

Generally, the religious beliefs and faith of these groups grew out of the natural environment and forces influencing their lives. Typically, there was an underlying belief that the spirit world was not set apart from life but was another stage of life. There are stories from native cultures of persons moving into a meditative state and letting go of life by collapsing their lungs through a specific breathing technique, or isolating themselves, drifting off on floating ice, or staying behind as their nomadic group moved on. The urgency of earthly participation and needs drove elders to move on, or in some cases perhaps to wander off and not return.

Where unique or odd behavior or functioning was believed to be a manifestation of spirit in a positive sense, not something feared or considered evil, and the community was thriving rather than just surviving, cultures were more inclusive of people suffering in this way and considering them "touched by God," direct mouthpieces to the ancestors. Their odd or unusual behavior was understood as a reaction to being sensitive to the threshold, or portal, between this material world and the spiritual realm. It was believed the threshold was thinner, more transparent, to those "touched" individuals, and made them operate in a different way. These oracles were treated with great respect, given latitude to function in their unique way, and supported by the community with shelter and sustenance.

Other cultures treated dementia with fear and ostracism. It makes me shudder to consider what some of the reactions to dementia have been over the ages. Severe situations probably ended swiftly because of the lack of resources or understanding to sustain someone with these issues.

Even in our modern era, in what we consider First World standards of living, there are circumstances in which lack of understanding, support, and resources can degrade a situation beyond repair. I often think of people with memory loss during natural disasters or national emergencies. For individuals with dementia in normal circumstances, there are greater and greater challenges to relate to the systems and routines we live by. We have all witnessed, through the media, examples of persons not cognitively impaired who make very poor decisions when under stress in unusual circumstances. How would someone with dementia manage such events? Who is looking out for them? And how many have we "lost" in chaotic times?

When societies are stable and thriving, there tends to be movement toward improving quality of life for citizens. Development doesn't just involve creating infrastructures for basic services; consideration of what's next occurs. What is that next evolutionary step society is taking? Examples are the treatment of women, children, and animals. The rights and treatment of these three groups immediately changes and/or improves when moving from a stressed culture to one that has more opportunities for repose. Looking at Western civilization today, recognition of issues of aging, both pro and con, has been evolving over the last two decades, especially with the baby boomer group reaching their retirement age. While ageism is still with us, counter forces resist stereotyping and raise the questions of how old is "old," and what does it really matter?

I run into what I call "dementia-ism" all the time—stereotyping and dismissal of persons with memory loss. Examples include:

- speaking in front of the person about them as if they are not there;
- a physician telling a family, "It's probably Alzheimer's," without doing any clinical or lab evaluations; or telling them they should contact hospice while the person with memory loss is still highly mobile, has a tan, and still hikes in the mountains with friends;
- an official saying all people with an Alzheimer's diagnosis should be in locked secure areas, with no acknowledgment of the stages of the process;
- staff or family helping too much and not allowing a person with memory loss to have a sense of ownership of their own day.

I could go on and on. I live in hope that dementia-isms will be replaced by more educated and compassionate interactions with those suffering memory loss, and that there will be a fundamental shift in how dementia is viewed in our culture. This is the cause that those of us in the field have rallied around for many years.

Throughout the book, you will hear me refer to "best practices" when discussing examples and stories that illustrate the process of dementia. These are the guiding principles of what we know today to be helpful, enlightened care approaches in dealing with memory loss.

Best practices in dementia care are based on the idea that the person is the most important factor to be considered in our actions. This focus on the individual guides how and why we do things a certain way. For example, we know in the middle stages of the dis-

ALZHEIMER'S DISEASE

Dr. Aloysius "Alois" Alzheimer was a physician in a large sanatorium in Germany at the turn of the last century. A young woman of 51, Auguste D., was admitted with all the signs of senility but, due to her age, she was felt to be far too young for this condition. Senility was thought to be a normal part of aging. The explanation was that somehow as people got older they had "senior moments" and would forget some things, might repeat stories, might become frailer, and might need more support from their families. Senility was increasing in frequency as the human lifespan lengthened, which led observers to conclude it must be an issue of aging.

Dr. Alzheimer was able to follow this case for a number of years, observing Auguste D. as she declined. When she died, he performed an autopsy and discovered significant cerebral pathologies that differentiated her condition from normal aging changes in the brain.

First, he found that there was excessive atrophy in Auguste D.'s brain. In a normal aging brain, some shrinkage of brain matter occurs, but in Auguste's case this was very pronounced. Next, compared with a healthy brain and its convoluted surface, the grooves had become very deep, and the inner portion of the brain where the ventricles are positioned had become hollowed out. There was also actual loss of brain matter. Another significant alteration was neurofibrillary tangles. The neural synapses were dying, tangling up, and in the process unable to send or absorb neural transmitter chemicals such as acetylcholine, which is essential for all levels of functioning. Lastly, Alzheimer noted amyloid plaques. In a normal aging brain there may be 3–15 of these plaques, which are made from a protein substance known as APoe-4. However, in a brain affected by this disease, there are so many plaques, they literally gum up the works. Think of a sticky, heavy, cholesterol-like substance laying itself out randomly on all parts of the brain. Alzheimer presented these findings at a conference in 1906, and the disease was named after him.

Currently, dementia is considered an umbrella term. We understand now that memory loss is not normal, no matter what the age. Although we may not understand all the causes or how to fix it, we know that this is caused by some kind of physical or chemical change and is truly aberrant.

ease that the person has difficulty initiating activities and that they have a short attention span; therefore, it is helpful to create a predictable structure to the day and pick things to do that genuinely interest the person with memory loss. Tapping into hobbies, skills, and talents the person always had is a much better place to start.

How we assist with the disease process and all the challenges that come up surrounding that person is based on the individual and what is going on for him or her at the time. Best practices combine tried-and-true principles that we know work with creativity in molding them for the specific situations that arise.

Between 1907 and the 1990s, science and medicine made some progress with tools to help diagnose dementia, of which Alzheimer's is the most prevalent of several forms. We now have CT and PET scans, MRI's, and functional assessment tools that give us more information about what the brain in a living person looks like and which symptoms can be categorized and viewed as common for certain diagnoses.

The Alzheimer's Association, the Alzheimer's Society, and other dementia advocacy groups have grown over the last 30 years. They function internationally, as well as in the United States. Their mission is to improve advocacy for persons with memory loss diagnosis and to support caregivers (both family members and professionals) by improving education and understanding of how to care for a person with these maladies. They also support increased funding for research efforts to find a cure or ways to help the disease plateau.

The Alzheimer's Association cautioned me not to record percentages for different dementias because they are constantly changing based on the research, and depending on what resource is used and when, the numbers can change. But to give some sense of the levels of occurrence, using the Alzheimer's Association's most recent numbers (2013), we can say today that 56 percent of all dementia diagnoses are of an Alzheimer's type, and 14–20 percent are considered vascular issues such as TIA's (transient ischemic attacks) or "mini-strokes" in lay terms. Individuals may have been compromised over a long period of time without outward symptoms. For example, the carotid arteries might be somewhat blocked, causing decreased profusion to the brain as well as other vascular issues that can cause dementing symptoms. Parkinson's, multiple sclerosis, AIDS, and lupus make up 8 percent of all dementia cases, while 4 percent are from brain injury, 12 percent are from multiple causes, and 6 percent are defined as "other."

The Alzheimer's Association was founded in 1980 to address the problem of families having loved ones being diagnosed with dementia but given no treatment or guidance on how to cope. People were told, "This is a chronic, progressive, degenerative, and debilitating disease of the brain, with gradual declines in intellectual ability, including memory, problem solving, and judgment. Eventually the disease leaves the person unable to care for themselves." Basically, the unintended message was, "Go home and wait for everything to unravel!" This was, of course, unacceptable.

Peter V. Rabins MD and Nancy Mace, a family member, wrote the first care guide for families, *The 36-Hour Day*, during those early days of the association in Chicago. This is still a practical and resourceful guide for families caring for a loved one at home.

FORMS OF DEMENTIA

The following information is available on the Alzheimer's Association website. Families coping with these forms of dementia can be assisted by some of the support, educational, and referral sources provided by the Alzheimer's Association.

Crutzfeldt-Jacob Disease (CJD) is a more rare, fatal brain disease caused by infection. Symptoms are failing memory, changes in behavior, and lack of muscular coordination. CJD progresses rapidly, usually causing death within a year.

Multi-Infarct Dementia (MID), also known as vascular dementia, results from brain damage caused by multiple strokes (infarcts) within the brain. Symptoms can include disorientation, confusion and behavioral changes. MID is neither reversible nor curable, but treatment of underlying conditions (e.g. high blood pressure) may halt progression.

Pick's Disease is a rare brain disease that closely resembles Alzheimer's, with personality changes and disorientation that may precede memory loss. Diagnosis is difficult and can only be confirmed by autopsy.

Frontal Lobe Dementia is a disease that causes a pronounced deterioration in the frontal lobe of the brain. It mimics Picks and Alzheimer's, with some symptoms causing personality changes and loss of inhibitions preceding memory loss.

Lewy Body Disease has been recognized only in recent years, but was presented by Dr. Lewy at the same 1907 conference as Dr. Alzheimer. Dr. Lewy identified specific lesions on the brain, hence the name Lewy body disease. The symptoms are a combination of Alzheimer's and Parkinson's disease. Usually, dementia symptoms are initially present, followed by the abnormal movements associated with Parkinson's. Other symptoms include hallucinations and delusions, falls, and varying consciousness. Persons with Lewy body can be very sensitive to psychotropic medications.

Huntington's Disease is an hereditary disorder characterized by irregular movements of the limbs and facial muscles, a decline in thinking ability, and personality changes. It can be positively diagnosed and symptoms controlled with drugs. Progression cannot be stopped.

Wernicke-Korsakoff Dementia is a chronic memory disorder caused by severe deficiency of thiamine (vitamin B-1). Korsakoff syndrome is most commonly caused by alcohol misuse, but certain other conditions like anorexia, AIDS, kidney dialysis, chronic infection, or cancer that spreads throughout the body, can cause it too. There are also genetic factors that can increase the predisposition to it.

My experience has been primarily with the Alzheimer's Association, since 1990, volunteering on the speaker's bureau, carrying out conference planning and developing trainings for our local chapter. It has grown from a grassroots organization, with each state and chapter having particular strengths and initiatives, to a nationally orchestrated force in the improvement of all areas of memory care.

Chapter 2

Then and Now
The Medical Model and Long-Term Care

My first employment as a newly graduated nurse was in a Catholic nursing home outside the city where I had attended school. The facility had been established by a charitable order of nuns focused on caring for the infirm. This building was a traditional structure, with long corridors and shiny nurses' stations and bustling staff in crisp white uniforms. "Patients," as we called them in those days, were divided by floors into groups based on levels of need and orientation. The third floor housed the greatest number of confused, memory-impaired elders. This floor was very chaotic and loud. Driving into the parking lot, one could actually hear them calling out.

Many of the core staff of nurses working there in 1983 had been inspired by the original group of nuns, so there was a great sense of tradition and mission. The street where the facility was located also led to the Catholic hospital, a kindergarten through 12th grade parochial school, a large church with parish structures, as well as regional administrative church offices. Having grown up in a Quaker household, I had never been exposed to the Catholic faith or to its rituals and ways of thinking. The setting was very rich with all these things.

The facility had a chapel on its second floor where mass was held daily in Latin. It was their practice at the time to broadcast the mass over the loudspeakers, giving those who could not attend in person the chance to participate by listening. Mass was being broadcast on my first day on the job. I found myself crushing pills with a metal device that made a loud banging noise to the tune of the sacred text—"Gloria Patri, et Filio, et Spiritu Sancto," (bang, bang, bang)—and all of that mixed with the sounds of the residents on the floor yelling, *AHH Ahhh!* The cacophony was unbelievable. This was truly a demented environment.

The unit had four ladies to a room, with 60 residents to the floor, and most had memory issues as well as other health concerns. We did not talk about Alzheimer's then—in those days, most people looked on memory loss as a part of aging—but this institutional model of care stripped patients of ways of expressing their individuality. Each four-person room contained a locker-sized closet for a few items of clothes, a bedside table with a couple of drawers, and a hospital bed for each patient. A curtain could be drawn between the beds, but there was no room for extra chairs in the room because of walkers, wheelchairs, and so on. If there were visitors, they found it difficult to visit in the patient's room. There was a common area, a lounge/dining room space, but it provided no privacy and had plastic furniture that was unappealing and completely institutional-looking.

Thankfully, today we have much better levels of service and ways to support people with a dementia diagnosis. But in 1983, many nursing homes cared for residents with Alzheimer's and other forms of dementia but had no special program or environments for them.

The medical model was driven primarily by staff needs and convenience and secondarily by patient needs—not by the broader level of needs we have as humans but by a belief that the medical needs are urgent and influence everything else. In a hospital this is relevant. In an acute, urgent situation, if you are bleeding to death, it doesn't matter that you have always loved animals or identified yourself strongly as a nurturing, stable mother, we have to find a way to stop your bleeding. But if you move to a long-term care facility fashioned on the medical model because you need more care and support than your current living situation can provide, as the months go by it matters less and less what fancy pills or therapy the place has to offer you if you are pining for your cat or dog, or your children don't stay and visit because the place doesn't allow or encourage casual, private family visiting.

This deprivation is magnified when someone has memory loss because nothing looks familiar and they often can't remember why they are there. They usually display a healthy level of vitality, and attempts at self-initiative can startle facility caregivers, because the care focused on physical disabilities and cognitive problems is a far second in the considerations of these settings.

What I observed at my first job was an inordinate amount of focus on keeping people safe and under control, which meant in many cases using chemical and physical restraints. This was abused in many settings. By limiting movement and expression of feelings, and not finding ways to channel this energy, caregivers essentially deadened it and hastened its disappearance. Many of these dear, classically demented people were pushed along the disease progression more rapidly by these negative approaches.

When I arrived at this facility, the director of nursing put me on this floor because of my background in special education and felt I could do well with these difficult patients. This was remarkably appropriate in my case. I heard later that everyone hated working that floor, so they always gave it to the newly hired nurse—but I was immediately hooked.

Many different layers of reality existed simultaneously. Residents were in various stages of dementia, and their moods, compounded by differing functional levels, created the atmosphere on "the ward," as they called it in those days. The personality, will, and sense of engagement of each patient were palpable presences. It felt totally wrong to me to have four women to a room. They had so little left from a lifetime of mothering large families or working in the world, and to have it all come down to this? All that life experience, all that uniqueness institutionalized because of needing some care?

There was, and still is in some facilities, a prejudice in favor of keeping confused, potentially agitated patients out of the way—away from view and the public. This often meant that, because they could not speak up for themselves, they got the worst living conditions with no access to the outdoors, and the environment was stripped of anything that could be moved or broken or bothered with. In order to look clean and medical (which in those days was supposed to be appealing and give the families confidence), facilities emphasized high-gloss tiles, washable paint and fluorescent lights, white sheets, white blankets, white bedspreads and towels, white privacy curtains, and molded plastic furniture.

Structured activities were not provided on the ward at that time, because health professionals still had not figured out that the challenging behaviors of their patients would lessen if they had things to do and ways of connecting to past roles and strengths. Residents had to fit into what was being offered in such a building and were taken where activities were being offered, based on their ability to participate. Since roughly 49 of the 60 residents on my floor were unable to participate in structured activities, it was a long day.

As a new nurse there was a lot for me to learn, from understanding the culture of the facility to providing the care each resident needed to managing the personalities of the nursing assistants. Some of the latter were 40 years older than me, so it felt strange to be their supervisor. I had to understand when to use their advice and when to make decisions based on my book learning. They soon got used to my odd ideas and vegetarian meals, as I got used to their old-salt wisdom.

WAKE UP!

One of the patients on my ward was an Italian-American woman from South Philadelphia. She was disoriented and would be quite agitated at times. She would slide down in her wheelchair and wave her arms in front of her face, calling out, "Maria! Maria Carvaggio!" when she wanted me. The first time she did this, I walked up to her and in my normal voice, with my regular accent, I responded politely, "How can I help you?" To which she responded by slapping me across the face.

Needless to say this was not what I expected, and it completely startled me. Retreating, I regrouped. The next time she called me, I replied with the best Italian accent I could muster, "Whadda ya want?" She reached for my hand and said, "I lova you!" What she was really saying when she slapped me was, "WAKE UP! You want to relate to me? You want to connect? You need to be recognizable in my world! You need to adjust to me!" It was a very valuable lesson.

One thing that quickly became apparent was the challenge of time. As the sole nurse on the floor, I used to add up the minutes: due to the required breaks, 60 patients on the ward, 7 hours per shift, meant 7 minutes per patient per work day. The caregivers had 15 elders to care for, which meant approximately 28 minutes per person for the work day. No wonder everyone felt time-pressured. Although the patients had no relation to linear or present time, they all needed time made for them. Budgets were (and are still) largely based on the time it takes to perform tasks physically—bathing, dressing, eating, taking pills, having treatments. Not how much time a resident with dementia needs in order to understand who they are, what they are doing, or why they are there. Nor how much time is needed to listen to them speak of their parent or to try to convince them they are meant to stay for dinner and not go home right now. All of the staff struggled with this issue.

An oriented resident in a long-term care facility realizes how to get someone's attention, how to get a need met, and that the caregiver is helping others. They know they are reliant on this person and tend to try not to frustrate or annoy this person. They may wish to be more demanding but sense they have to juggle their own wishes when working with the caregiver. Someone with dementia, however, will often have difficulty with this specific issue because they don't remember you just helped them or just interacted with them.

They won't realize they have undone something, for instance, when you just helped them dress and they have undressed again. Budgets have to reflect time to be human with one another as well as time to get physical things done. With dementia folks this often means time to do it all over again as well.

A SNOWY NIGHT

One evening, a winter storm blew in and we had multiple staff calling in to say that they were unable to get to work. It meant that those of us who had worked the evening shift had no replacements and we had to stay over.

I was already pretty tired from the week, and it was around 3 a.m. I noticed I was feeling different, somehow altered; it's hard to describe. I was walking down the darkened corridor when suddenly the walls seemed to melt away. I could see each person lying in their bed, and there was a silver cordlike light emanating from each person's torso toward the ceiling, which also somehow wasn't there. The patients who felt the least connected to Earth, who had the frailest bodies, or who had minds that were not connected to the here and now had the strongest most vibrant lights flowing toward the heavens. Those patients that were connected to the present, who were very much active participants in their day-to-day lives, had threadlike, less vibrant emanations.

An oriented resident in a long-term care facility realizes how to get someone's attention, how to get a need met, and that the caregiver is helping others. They know they are reliant on this person and tend to try not to frustrate or annoy this person. . . . Someone with dementia, however, will often have difficulty with this specific issue because they don't remember you just helped them or just interacted with them.

I found myself continuing to walk along the darkened hall, but now the walls were back in place. Whatever this experience was, it was very quick and made me wonder if I was sleepwalking and somehow dreaming. But the image stayed with me and caused me to question what was actually going on here. Were the residents who seemed so disconnected actually unavailable because their hearts and minds were experiencing a deeper, more vital connection to the realm of spirit than to this earthly plane? Were they busily at work in a deep meditative way while we were so entrenched in our perception of our reality that we couldn't see it?

I had heard that sleep allows for restoration and revitalization to occur at many levels, that REM sleep and dreaming are crucial to maintaining one's stability and mental health. Sleep is also a time that allows the spirit to work more deeply in individuals. For those who believe in angelic influence, one's Angel or Higher Self dips down in the form of dreams and is able to plant seeds that after we awaken are able to germinate and provide inspiration and direction. How often do you hear of people "sleeping on it" and waking up with a decision. Is it really just us, or are we getting some help?

Prayer is another more conscious form of this connection: praying before sleep, letting things go to a higher source and stating, "Thy will be done." Acting in the daylight on the prayers posted at night has enabled many to stay on higher ground in the midst of tough situations. Again, are we getting help? I believe we are. This help may be coming from a higher power or source, but it can also be directed or provided by others in our human community.

A great deal of research has been done in recent years on the power of prayer and healing. For example, in situations where individuals know each other, such as in families, and ask their local prayer groups to pray at a bedside, improvements in patient outcome have been documented. Measurable improvements in patient outcomes have also been documented in long-distance prayer situations, regardless of whether the participants knew the person they were praying for. We also do not know at what level a prayer has been received. We often look for relief in the physical symptom we are trying to ease, but there may be an easing on an emotional level, or some other level of self that is hidden from outside observers.

On a simple biological level, studies have shown that if a red blood cell is prayed for while blood is being drawn, when it is dropped in saline solution it will resist the inevitable bursting that occurs in saline solution, whereas a red blood cell that is not prayed for bursts immediately on contact with the solution.

There is a saying that, "When babies are born, humans rejoice and angels cry, but when humans die, angels rejoice and humans cry." I believe that when we die, those who loved us and have gone on ahead are there to greet us and welcome us home; dying is the inevitable step.

But to have an illness and have to live in an altered way can be very challenging for the person dealing with the condition. I believe that when we are taking a longer transitioning process, following chronic or terminal diagnosis, loving beings—angels—support us, comfort us, visit us, and serve as companions in this life prior to our exit. We don't see them, partly because most of us have had this extrasensory ability trained out of us at a very early age by our culture.

For example, I once met a mother whose three-year-old child had reported spending time with the family dog and accurately described her grandparents on numerous occasions, including what the visit entailed and what was said. He had never met the dog or her grandparents, though, because they had all passed long before his birth. This frightened the mother, but an elder, a wise woman within her family circle, felt that this was very special, not something to be scared of but to be encouraged, and that this child was blessed. I think the mother felt conflicted, trying to reconcile old beliefs based on science with new beliefs. Also, this was not part of her own experience—the family dog and grandparents had never visited her. I think her overriding preference was that she wished that this was not happening and that her son would stop having visits . . . and certainly would stop talking about it. This attitude seems to be very common in our modern-day lives.

Some cultures do not do this. They appreciate that the maya (world of illusion) we call "reality" isn't really there in the way we imagine it is. In Thailand, for example, they believe that spirits inhabit and share spaces with humans. If someone builds a house or a building, a small spirit house is also built on the property in order to honor and give refuge to the spirits that live there, too. The visible and invisible coexist.

When I think of this belief, it makes me feel as if the air must be thick with spirits, that it almost has mass, like water, and we are moving though spirit in every waking moment. We might even be sloshing through spirit. It's a beautiful and comforting image. The other reason many of us don't see or sense these things is that we are so busy going about the work of our lives. It's as if we each made a commitment to participate in this reality and use it as classroom for our learning. That requires a certain amount of engagement with the "reality" we have mutually agreed to in order to accomplish these experiences.

When people have Alzheimer's disease, they cannot hold onto the mundane aspects of life that have the rest of us in their grip, utterly distracted by reality. They have slowly let go, not willingly but inevitably, of all the business of living. They have moved deeply into memory, and beyond.

Very early in my nursing career, I began questioning the instruction to set people straight about their delusions and hallucinations. Many patients see their long-gone family members and have visits and speak about it later. Some say they are going to go talk to their parents, then come back saying that they have. So who am I to say that this hasn't really happened? Just because I can't see these deceased family members doesn't mean they aren't there.

I once had a resident who had momentary deathlike seizures/strokes that lasted about 10 minutes. She would go completely gray. We couldn't find a pulse initially. She was not breathing, and just when we thought we were going to have to call 911, she would take a deep breath and start pinking up. Within a half hour, she was walking, talking, and back to her old self.

We contacted the daughter about the episodes each time one occurred, and she started noting a curious pattern. The episodes were occurring on important family dates, such as wedding anniversaries, kids' birthdays, and her husband's birthday. After the episodes, this resident would say things like, "I had to talk to my husband. I had some questions I wanted to ask my husband. He always made good sense to me. We had a nice long chat."

When people have Alzheimer's disease, they cannot hold onto the mundane aspects of life that have the rest of us in their grip, utterly distracted by reality. They have slowly let go, not willingly but inevitably, of all the business of living. They have moved deeply into memory, and beyond.

The resident's husband had passed away some time earlier, but her sense of him living in her longer-term memory was more immediate to her than her current life and living situation. We all believed—both family and staff—that she really was having conversations with her husband. She just went out "excarnating," instead of the lightweight version of dream encounters. We also knew that one day she would go out and not return.

Returning now to the story about the first facility I worked in . . .

The director of nursing approached me one day and stated, "You are very philosophical. I want you to take the evening nurse position on the third-floor pavilion." This felt like a unique opportunity—a Quaker girl caring for 14 priests—and I agreed to the change.

Many things on this floor turned out to be different from the floor I had first worked on. For starters, it was very quiet—so quiet, in fact, that when visitors came to the floor, they would whisper, "Sister Megan, is Father So-and-So here?" To which I would reply,

"Yes. He is in room such-and-such. We don't need to whisper. I'm a nurse, not a nun, so you can just call me Megan."

I also received a lot of blessings from the priests, which was very touching. I didn't realize priests drank alcohol, and I had no experience of hard liquor. I had to ask the director of nursing what was meant by "scotch on the rocks," and, indeed, "What are rocks?" which brought great teasing for a few weeks. Most of the priests had cocktails before their evening medications. It felt strange to be making all those drinks wearing my white cap and dress and passing them out on a tray.

A number of priests on the wing had dementia. Father B. had spent his life teaching in boys' schools. He had giant blue eyes and would sometimes hallucinate that the boys had invaded the rectory. I had never experienced hallucinations like his. I had to participate in shushing the boys out of the dayroom. He would say, "No, no, over there! Oh good! Wait! There is one more." Once I got them all out, he would be so relieved.

He also spent most of his time stripping, which I understand now is a very common dementia behavior. The staff had created an ingenious maze of safety pins to attach his vest restraint (worn because of frequent falls) to his clothes. He would say things like, "Hail, Mary, full of grace," as he worked each safety pin, and when he got each one loose would throw it away with a "Praise the Lord" or "Amen" and go on to the next pin, until he was completely naked. We would approach him and ask, "Father B., can I help you get dressed?" He would respond, "Bless you, my child. Yes, yes, that would be helpful," and happily get dressed again, patiently waiting for all the pins to be found and fastened. Then he would start all over again.

Father D. would sit in the recliner in his room and quietly hallucinate all day that he was revisiting all the wonderful ceremonies in which he had officiated. He had a strange sense of time. If I had to disturb him, I would whisper why I was doing so in his ear (medicine, a meal), and he'd say, "Not yet," or "Not now. We haven't finished the christening," or "He is about to take his vows." He would then give me a time to come back—20 minutes, 10 minutes, half an hour. When I returned at the time he had stated, he would be ready. This gentleman was completely blind. It was very touching to me that he was able to spend his time enjoying the beautiful images of his active past.

Father R. was not disoriented but was a diabetic on dialysis. He and I became fast friends. I would share my dinner with him, and he would give me catechism lessons. We had great discussions about God and faith, religion, death and dying, Quakerism versus Catholicism, difference and similarities, about angels, raising families, teaching children, travel, and all other aspects of our lives at that time.

He was the one who first told me the classic joke that apparently is altered by inserting different faiths depending on who is telling it. In his version, though, the joke involved a Protestant dying and going to Heaven who noticed a huge wall in one area. He asked St. Peter about it, and St. Peter said, "Oh, that's because the Catholics think they are the only ones up here."

Father R. had a rich sense of humor, as well as a strong faith. He decided to facilitate catechism. I needed to bring a question to him every week and he would open Vatican 2 and we would discuss it. At one point, I remember him throwing his arms up and sighing about my questions, stating that he had not had questions like that before, and just shook his head.

During this period, I also had many dreams about working for Mother Teresa in India. I would be in the sari of the order, hand-feeding a dying person reclined on a grass mat in a hot, humid, darkened area. All around me in this simple, somewhat crowded area, others were quietly bustling and receiving care. Father R. and I went round and round about these dreams. He felt it was a sign I needed to become a nun and work with this great teacher. I felt it was some kind of parallel reality that I was experiencing. I really loved these animated and thoughtful discussions with this dear religious, faithful, and open man. We continued to correspond until his death in 1987.

I had read Florence Nightingale's book, *Notes on Nursing*, prior to attending nursing school. I was struck by how much common sense the British founder of modern nursing had had back then, during the Victorian period and the Crimean War, and also that the role of nurse was all-encompassing. In Florence Nightingale's day, the nurse (always a woman) cooked the meal, fed the patient, and treated their wounds. She helped them exercise, created diversional activities, spent time listening, and did the laundry.

In the modern era, we have parceled all these aspects of care to different departments and specialists. Dietary does the cooking, Housekeeping cleans; Laundry launders. Physical Therapy focuses mainly on the legs and mobility; Occupational Therapy focuses on the upper extremities and tasks of daily living; Nursing helps with medications and treatment; and Activities provides programs. The necessity for this approach is often determined by the numbers of patients the staff is trying to serve. A strongly functioning team can provide care in a seamless way, even if there are many departments that provide all the different aspects of care.

On the other hand, this approach can create fragmentation, placing on the patient the burden of making sense of how everything works and who is who—something that, with dementia, is impossible. Additionally, it can cause a distancing from the aspects of daily life that bring some measure of grounding in ordinary reality, and that can further impair a person's sense of dis-ease.

Florence Nightingale, OM, RRC (1820–1910) was a celebrated English social reformer and statistician, and the founder of modern nursing. She came to prominence while serving as a nurse during the Crimean War, where she tended to wounded soldiers.

For example, in hospitals someone delivers meal trays. That person may see a diet order and check the plate against what the order is, but they might not realize the person needs more assistance. The nurse, pulled away caring for other patients, may not realize the food tray has been delivered. The person in a later stage of Alzheimer's is unable to open containers, plastic silverware wrappers, or even realize there is something under the plastic lid. A different person returns to pick up the food and notices it's untouched. Many people in the hospital are ill enough to have their appetite affected, so they do not think to notify the nurse or ask questions. I have had patients lose 6–15 pounds during a short hospital stay, then discovered that they were never assisted in simple meal setup. The only thing that had kept them alive and hydrated was their intravenous hookup.

A SOCIAL MODEL OF CARE

Since the early 1970s, there have been movements in long-term care to promote a social model of care and to individualize the treatment of elders in care settings. Some of this was prompted by the civil rights movement and looking at the rights of elders in institutionalized care. The Gray Panthers brought greater awareness to the plight of elders in settings where previously their voices had not been heard. In a social model of care, the main theme is "person-centered care." The person's individuality, social history, and current interests and needs drive and inform the kind of activities, support, and care the person receives. The residence or facility involves elders in all aspects of the organization—for example, including them in interviewing potential new hires. A social model wants the facility to respond to the needs and wishes of the people who live there when it comes to hiring staff, making house rules, developing menus, activities, and so forth.

One early long-term care movement was the Live Oak Tree project, Pioneer Network, which in the 1990s, evolved into the Culture Change movement, with matching momentum coming from Dr. William Thomas, founder of The Eden Alternative. The Eden Alternative has developed extensive training programs and certifies facilities, in order to assist long-term care facilities in making the shift from a medical model to a social model. The Eden Alternative also continues the relationship with facilities on specific points to help them maintain certification and the integrity of the program.

Another approach in a social model of care involves the use of what are known as "global workers" or "universal staff." This does not mean that the facility is hiring people from all over the world—although that might be the case; it means that they are pulling back different areas of function in the residence within the scope of fewer individuals. The same staff helps with laundry, meal service, and dressing, grooming, bathing, activities, and medications. The role encompasses all these duties. This maximizes continuity and familiarity with all aspects of the patient's day and experiences and matches changing needs. This approach is particularly advantageous to a person with memory loss.

A parallel movement in hospital settings has been developed by an organization called Planetree. It was started by a patient who felt her experience in a hospital in the 1970s was far from therapeutic and healing. She raised awareness and created a momentum to develop training, goals, and guidelines that are voluntarily adopted with this model of patient-centered care. Hospitals began to recognize that this approach improved the patients' experiences, as well as meeting their own internal measurements of quality improvement, reducing turnover, error rates, and so on.

The Planetree model permits patients to see their own chart, for example, plus encourages hospitals to design their patient areas to be more soothing and friendly; reviews meal plans and how to improve their nutritional value and presentation; and helps staff remember to take time to refresh their own batteries during very difficult, high-paced work. Planetree is now partnering with provider networks, moving from hospitals into rehab and long-term care settings as well. All are part of a growing worldwide network of organizations certified in the Planetree approach, and continually working toward improving care and everyone's experience while giving or receiving it.

For over 40 years, individuals and companies in the senior healthcare industry have been diligently working on improving living environments, staff training and family support, as well as activities and other programs for residents, so I find it sad that there is still so much inertia in this field. Those of us who are "envelope pushers," the shakers and rollers, want this type of living situation to be equal to home or choosing a new apartment. One should be able to list the pros and cons the same way one does in other living situations:

- "This apartment has two bedrooms, a full kitchen, and a nice living space with a porch."
- "This apartment includes meals that I can get in their main dining area, but I still have my own kitchen I can use when I want to."
- "This apartment gives me access to meal service, transportation, a communal garden and greenhouse, chaplain services, and social events, and there is a nurse here I can contact with concerns as well as caregiver assistance in the morning and evening."
- "This place has a kitchen I can cook in when I want to, and also a place where my grandkids can play when they visit."
- "I like my privacy, but that place has people who can help me, and sometimes I feel lonely and overwhelmed."
- "This place has regular social opportunities, and living alone I don't get that."

Being able to make choices is so much better than being terrified of being put in a nursing home, fearful that death will quickly occur, or dreading the impending doom of many long days and nights in a place that smells of urine, is devoid of family contact, and has routines that look nothing like the pattern the elder previously had. There are too many facilities in America that still feel this way.

This is a two-fold issue. First, facilities are only as isolated as their communities make them. A facility or residence may be doing all the right things, but it can't do everything. No matter what the resources are for a setting, whether private pay or Medicaid, it can't be all things to all people. It needs a flow of individuals from the surrounding community who participate in the life there. Families continue to play a crucial role. Volunteers connecting and spending one-to-one time with someone can make an enormous difference to a person's sense of place and belonging. We are happy to see all the visitors during holiday seasons, but there are vacant times in the rest of the year.

Second, we need to keep building the bridges of normalcy between the "outside" community and the "inside" world of a long-term care community. We need to create a welcoming environment that puts visitors at ease, provides areas to chat privately, allows

"One of our residents moved into our facility because she was reclusing at home and refusing to go out. The family was extremely agitated about moving her in, being absolutely certain that she would be very upset. On the contrary, she was thrilled to be here, thought it was a lovely place, and never missed a beat. She soon became a constant companion for one of our male residents who had recently lost his wife. They lived here for several years, were constant companions, attended all activities together, except for worship service, which she loved and he preferred not to attend."

— Judy Dickinson
Concierge and Master Gardener
Program Coordinator

pets and children a place to play, and ways for children or adults to easily participate in whatever is currently occurring in the facility.

We must get rid of the old stereotype of visitors being overwhelmed by odors as they enter a long-term care center, of viewing "parked" residents languishing in hallways scattered among scary equipment, and disconnected staff bustling about or not visible. It's fine for someone to need a rest, but if this person is resting in a soft seating area, in a normally scaled living room, it feels very different from leaning to one side in a wheelchair that is slightly faced toward a wall in a cluttered hallway. If the person resting is near others when they wake up, they feel comforted by their presence; when they awaken in a hall looking at a wall, this is alienating and dehumanizing. Some architects and designers make the mistake of not making spaces big enough to accommodate the number of wheelchairs routinely used in these settings nor providing enough furniture for transfer opportunities.

In memory care units, staff have to remain open and approach visitors to assess their comfort and what added information might be most helpful. Because the activity level in a memory care unit can be higher, and along with it the potential for more interactions with different resident behaviors, advising visitors on what to expect can help them feel more comfortable and able to cope, especially if something unexpected occurs. For example, they may encounter an elder who thinks they are a long-lost family member or an elder who is difficult to understand, using nonsensical words. Offering the visitor some guidance on ways to respond to situations like this will go a long way toward helping them feel comfortable with this "new normal."

> I found a friend today.
>
> Her Name is Mary.
>
> She might not tell you her name,
> but if you silently say Mary,
> she raises her head to present her
> bright eyes and lovely smile.
>
> She might say "have a nice
> day," or "nice meeting you,"
> or sing a song.
>
> Mary is loved by her family,
> daughter, and friends.
>
> She is graced to live at Balfour.
>
> For me to volunteer here
> is an honor; one receives more
> than you give.
>
> I found a friend today.
>
> — Diane Lawrence, volunteer,
> with Visiting Therapy dogs, Daisy
> and Winston

Once, I was doing an exit interview with a wonderful young caregiver with whom I had worked for almost four years. She was moving out of state, and I asked her what she had learned from this job, how had she grown. She sat quietly for a moment and said, "Older people are no different from any of us. People with dementia are no different from us. They all, we all, have the same feelings and needs. They want to laugh and be silly, they want to be listened to and be taken seriously, they want to be reassured and loved, they want to love and be helpful, make a contribution, just like everyone else. I learned that here."

It was one of the reasons she did so well with this job. Her role was that of peership. Yes, she provided care, and accomplished tasks with great skill. But this underlying stance was touchingly visible in her interactions with the residents, and it was wonderful to hear her voice it so clearly.

"One day I was sitting chatting with Marianne, a resident who had worked in the field of psychology. As we chatted, I mentioned how I wanted to be a psychologist and how disappointed I was that the college I was going to emphasized experimental psych, not behavioral. I told her I wasn't interested in working with rats.

She looked me straight in the eye and said, 'Oh, you were fortunate, then.'

I responded, imagining she was talking about my decision of behavioral psyche over experimental psych, 'How so?'

Marianne said, 'That would not have been a good fit for you. You would have found that out later.'

Curious, I continued, 'What do you mean, Mary?'

She quickly said, 'A psychologist is a passive listener; you, on the other hand, have so much exuberance and joy, you would not have been able to express your true gifts.'

Her clarity shocked me. Her ability to see the incongruence so acutely brought me to a powerful place of emotional honesty and self-acceptance. I thanked her for her honesty and insight. She smiled. I quietly sat with her, enjoying the intimacy we now shared."

— Phyllis, Life Enrichment (Activities) Coordinator

Chapter 3

....

Introduction to a
Philosophical Stance

Growing up, I was taught that we all have higher selves, and that this aspect of self is aware of far more than our everyday self. Through our dreams, meditation, and moments of inspiration, we strengthen our sense of knowing. We can access and work with ever greater consciousness with the higher self. I was taught that in life, we are meant "To learn, to love, and to make a difference." This has been the foundation of my perspective.

My mother would say that the world is actually perfect. I would be on some rant as a teenager about crime, poverty, or disease, and I would say, "How can that be? This or that is terrible!" She would respond, "It causes a sense of immediacy, a mobilization responding to whatever the situation is. There are constant opportunities to learn and to make a difference everywhere you look." She also defined evil in two ways: "That which is misunderstood" or "Mid-point in a changing good." These two definitions have been very helpful to me.

My mother was actively working toward and achieved the glistening ability to love unconditionally. It radiated from her during the last couple of years before she died. She was a very compassionate person, but this was earned and exercised in the context of a life that had had many wonderful opportunities but also had had many hard and wrenching experiences that she had worked to transform. You will hear her voice often in what I write. My parents, both wise, always kept an open hand with me. They gave me many things to think about, but ultimately always felt I should test these theories out for myself, figure out what was true for me—my truth. This has been a great blessing.

When I speak of Spirit, I mean that divine aspect in each of us that is connected to a greater understanding, a greater knowing that flows into a greater divinity. It is not tied to a specific faith or religion, although in our day-to-day practices and experiences we may resonate to a specific belief, and this assists us in remembering this foundational aspect of our lives. Religion is a cultural magnification of a deeper spiritual understanding, which through outward ritual creates communal resonance.

Religion is a reassuring structure, but it defeats its highest ideal when it limits and condemns. It is human to wish all things to be black and white, good or evil, so that one can be in a blessed state and perceive others to be in a hellish state, somehow outside the realm of God's consideration or protection. I do not feel this attitude is a manifestation of God's wrath but a human desire for judgment and retribution. Spirit appears to me to be infinitely spacious, encompassing more than I will ever be able to perceive or comprehend on my own.

Here are two teaching stories that have been very significant to me.

Many years ago, I read the book *God's Pauper: St. Francis of Assisi* by the Greek writer Nikos Kazantzakis. In this story about St. Francis, Kazantzakis uses the voice of Brother Leo, St. Francis's companion, to describe the events as they unfold. As we discover, Brother Leo is a regular kind of guy, with basic wishes and desires, but who also realizes there is something extraordinary about Francis. Brother Leo wishes they would not have to sleep outside in the rain, or could have gotten some stew in the last town. He thinks prayer is a good idea, and being charitable is essential, but he has a more normal, sane approach to things.

The reader feels the tension between what makes a person insane, extreme in their behaviors and ideas, versus divinely inspired and acting from an alignment with something that is beyond our normal considerations. Brother Leo wrestles with this throughout the story.

In one incident, they discuss how difficult it is to decipher God's will in their lives. Francis, who fears lepers, has not slept all night following a conversation they had had regarding understanding God's will. He arises hurriedly in the morning and wakes Brother Leo, saying, "I must embrace the next leper we come across and kiss him on the mouth."

Brother Leo is imploring Francis to reassess the meaning of this message and escape from this task when they hear the tinkling of the leper's bell approaching from a distance. Terrified but determined, Francis starts striding in the direction of the bell, with Brother Leo in hot pursuit. The leper sees them and starts ringing his bell frantically to warn them to stay away. Realizing Francis is undeterred and still fast approaching, the leper lets out a cry and collapses in a heap.

The leper has only stumps for fingers, half his nose is missing, and his lips are an oozing wound. Francis grabs him in a deep embrace, kisses him, and begins to carry him toward the town. After walking a distance, Francis suddenly bends over, opens the robe he had wrapped the leper in, and finds the leper has completely disappeared! Francis cannot speak for a time and is overcome, weeping. Finally he turns to Brother Leo and states, "What I understood: all lepers, cripples, sinners, if you kiss them on the mouth . . . they all become Christ."

What opens up in us when we embrace that which causes us to recoil? What grows in our hearts when we face some dark aspect of ourselves or perceive in others? My mother often commented that under every angry emotion or feeling of hate was fear, and under every fear was a need for understanding and love.

The second story is a true story of an experience I had while living in Scotland in a Camphill community for handicapped individuals. What amazed me was the coincidence of reading about St. Francis three months earlier and then witnessing the following events in our nearest Scottish town.

In this town, there was a man who would go to the local grocery/café on his days off from his sheltered workshop in Camphill. He would enjoy his favorite coffee cake, then proceed to stand outside the front door for the rest of the day. Standing there, he would greet each person stopping in at the store with great exuberance, holding his hand out to be shaken.

Let's remember to greet the light in each other and hold to that feeling, because it is more real than what we think real is.

The challenge was that he had a very deformed hand, so each greeting was an opportunity to overcome our antipathy, overcome aversion, and reach out in response to the humanity in this person. When folks responded and shook his hand and warmly greeted him back, it was like the sun was shining all around the two people in the moment of interaction. And it continued to shine as each went their separate ways. His glee was absolute.

However, with people who could not overcome their shock at seeing the hand, their recoiling and avoiding eye contact caused pure disappointment. He was not judgmental or self-conscious, just extraordinarily sad. The missed opportunity was so glaring.

He seemed to be the town crier, whose message was: "Go deeper. Go beyond the material world, the obvious. Let's remember to greet the light in each other and hold to that feeling, because it is more real than what we think real is."

....

Chapter 4

What I Understand
About "Dis-ease"

When I was growing up, our family physician, Dr. Henry N. Williams, was an interesting and unique individual, as well as a devoted doctor who made house calls and also served families in the Amish community. He was a true believer in the holistic model of care and was not afraid to look at all resources when trying to assist patients in their healing. After graduating from medical school he became interested in homeopathy and eventually became the president of The Homeopathic Society. He believed in hands-on healing and the power that resided in the patient to "heal thyself."

Dr. Williams was also a very good clinician, and would make decisions with each patient on what resources to use in their care. I never detected any conflict between using allopathic approaches (modern medications, antibiotics, and so on) or homeopathic or herbal approaches. Different situations called for different approaches. He understood when there was a need to swiftly treat and clear something out of the body and when to allow a slower process, so that the body could fight and clear something out under its own means with gentler support.

As an eight-year-old sick with some "bug," I can remember Dr. Williams asking me, as he listened to my lungs, "Why do you think you need to be sick?" I couldn't answer him then, but I knew that every time I wasn't feeling okay this question was going to come up. I started considering it myself, and sometimes I did have a sense of some of the dynamics that contributed to an increased vulnerability in my body that made it easier for a bug to take hold.

Louis Pasteur and fellow scientist Claude Bernard, two giants of 19th-century biology, had an ongoing argument about the nature of germs and their effects on health. Pasteur firmly believed in germs. They were out there, and they could get us, so we had to do certain things to avoid their ill effects, such as "pasteurizing" milk. His colleague, on the other hand, firmly believed it was the "soil"—the condition of the host that the germ landed on—that created the dynamic of illness. Why do some people get sick during a flu epidemic and others do not? Why did 13 million people die during the Black Death, and yet Europe is still populated? This argument went on until, as the legend goes, Pasteur lying on his deathbed blurted out, "You are right! It is the Soil!" and promptly died.

This age-old argument continues today. On the one hand, we have the modern medicine of the last 200-plus years, which believes very strongly in what can be proven, repeated, and studied on a physical level. We also have approaches to medicine from other cultures all over the globe by which humanity has steered its course and survived for thousands of years.

Practices fall in and out of favor, or are revived for different purposes. For example, we know today, thankfully, that blood-letting typically does not heal a lot of patient woes. Even so, leeches have gone from being the answer, to being vilified, to being increasingly valued today in wound debridement (cleansing) and healing. Leeches, it turns out, produce a chemical that stops the host's blood from clotting at the site of attachment, thereby giving researchers studying them new options in the development of anticoagulant medications.

Traditional Chinese medicine (TCM), which is over 5,000 years old, utilizes a number of healing modalities, one of which is acupuncture, a technique that involves small needles being inserted at specific points along energy lines, or meridians, on the surface of the body to treat certain ailments. Western medicine scoffed at this approach until someone finally did some research and was able to prove to themselves that it actually did help with certain conditions, such as pain and arthritis.

The arrogance that is played out in the realm of treatment is maddening to me. If you break your arm, yes, the emergency room is very helpful. But if you have lost your way in some other part of yourself, a "fix" may involve a very different path of treatment.

Healers and shamans of various cultures have been aware that some illnesses relate to spiritual distress, some relate to relational distress, and some are really what you ate last night. Sometimes an illness requires adding an ingredient to the person's body, or it requires purging or expunging something. Sometimes a whole ritual is required, and the shaman must go into an altered state to accompany the person in another realm through a process to get into better balance. Sometimes they simply make a specific tea, and that is adequate.

In the Western approach, the field of psychiatry has had to fight very hard for legitimacy over the last 100 years, and it too has made mistakes and grown in its approaches to care. Psychiatrists no longer blast schizophrenics with fire hoses to get them to stop being delusional, yet at one time we accepted that as "treatment." Western medical doctors felt women should be knocked unconscious to deliver babies and that they shouldn't breast feed. Now they don't feel that way. Somehow, we as individuals have to navigate all this and take personal responsibility in regards to our own health, how we want to be treated, what we want to be treated with, and how our personal beliefs come into play as we consider treatment possibilities.

Dr. Williams, our family doctor in Pennsylvania, was also the medical director for a local residential school for disabled children, Camphill Special School. Through him and this school I became aware of Anthroposophy, an esoteric philosophy and spiritual movement founded by Austrian social reformer Rudolf Steiner that led to the development of the Waldorf method of education. Camphill was part of a network of communities for handicapped children and adults based on Steiner's Waldorf method, and modified to meet special needs individuals since the Second World War. The original school/community had begun on an estate in Scotland called Camphill, hence the name. In time, they were invited by families around the world to bring this life experience to special individuals in many new locations.

I was one of those nontraditional students who did well in school if I was interested, but somehow got distracted, couldn't focus, and didn't care, if I wasn't interested. This caused a lot of stress to my dear, brilliant, traditionally learning parents and older sister. Each semester brought conversations in my father's study along the lines of, "Megan, do you want to be a waitress the rest of your life?" Not that waitressing was a bad gig, but education is a big part of having choices later. I would feel these big steel doors closing slowly, creaking, then BAM! No future for Megan!

It was Dr. Williams who suggested that maybe I should spend a year living and working in this community with special children. I have a special sister I love very much, who taught and continues to teach me a great deal about life. Dr. Williams knew this, of course, and felt I would be a natural with these kids. My parents and he felt it would give me a year to grow up a little and perhaps sort out what I was truly interested in pursuing, which at that point I thought was art or psychology.

Suffice it to say, the Camphill experience truly could be a whole additional book! Not only did I go there that first year after high school, I stayed three more years. I ended up completing the "curative course," which, in essence, is a Waldorf special education approach. This time in my life was very rich and meaningful to me. It was life altering and continues to be a reference point and resource in my work today.

During my time at Camphill, each of us "dorm parents" was assigned a group of children (usually three severely disabled children of about the same age) to care for during the traditional school year. During the holiday, these children would return home to their families, and each summer a new group would be assigned for the next school year. This setup gave us the opportunity to be involved with and learn about various children and

RUDOLF STEINER

Rudolf Steiner was a prolific writer and speaker and had a following of individuals from various walks of life who began developing areas of activity according to their own interests, using his guidance and instruction. Although he died in 1925, his anthroposophical work continues and has grown into a worldwide movement in medicine, education, agriculture, the arts, communities, and schools. Private individuals can be found working diligently today on the principles he laid out, furthering research and therapies, and experiencing an alternative life style that harkens back in many ways to a slower-paced, more natural way of living as practiced by earlier generations.

their challenges. Caring for these children was a 24-hour-a-day job, six and a half days a week. We had just one afternoon off a week, during which time another staff member would take responsibility for our charges.

During the week, we would ready the children for their day and provide assistance with grooming, bathing, dressing, meals, housekeeping, and laundry. The staff involved in the training program—at that point a three- to four-year educational program, would then head off to their scheduled classes or help in various programs throughout the community. Sheltered workshops added opportunities such as weaving, bakery, pottery, candle-making, woodworking, gardening, and, in the adult communities, dairy production, animal husbandry, and biodynamic farming. Some dorm parents assisted in the classrooms or with various therapy programs.

The beauty of this therapeutic environment was the acknowledgment that each person makes a contribution.

The community had a very strong rhythm and structure. This manifested in daily routines as well as seasonal cycles and celebrations. The daily routine had periods of high activity and interaction, followed by periods of rest and reduced activity. This pattern of expansion and contraction was repeated throughout the day. Having all gone in various directions after breakfast, we would return to our residence for lunch, which was the main meal of the day, again assisting our charges. Then a one-hour rest period was provided, after which we all headed back in our different directions. We returned to our households for dinner, where we would assist our dorm children with evening activities and going to bed.

Families with children lived in the same households as coworkers and groups of special needs children all around the property. This formed the nucleus of the Camphill community. Various special events, plays, festivals, worship services, dances, weddings, and christenings, all focused on seasonal changes or needs, took place throughout the year. Together, they helped strengthen the framework of experiences we had together. There was nothing institutional about these homes and communities, which were placed in tranquil settings among woods and farmlands. It was the social model to an extreme, and everyone took their turn doing different chores. For some people, living this way can be a wonderful way to develop their abilities; for others, it presents challenges. As always in the world, there are imperfections in human ventures and things to be learned from each other.

The beauty of this therapeutic environment was the acknowledgment that each person makes a contribution. In assessing what tasks needed to be completed there was an understanding that every person could play a part, based on their abilities and unique talents. It was clear that by involving everyone, each person had ownership or an experience of relating to the stuff of daily life. Things were not being done *to* or *for* the special residents but *with* them. This immediately changed the paradigms of who is ill, who is the patient, who is the caregiver, and who is the victim in some sad circumstance. It's both ennobling and normalizing. For example, when we were washing dishes, one child would scrape the plate's contents into the compost bucket, one would scrub, one would rinse, one would dry, and one would put them away.

With our individual challenges, we each formed an unusual family. In one household, for example, Richard, a tall autistic boy, would take the compost to the heap at the upper gardens after dinner each night. A staff person had accompanied him many times until he was able to do this on his own. He enjoyed the evening sky and walks through the woods and being greeted by other households as he passed by on both parts of the trip. It was very helpful to his household, the gardener appreciated his additions to the soil, and Richard knew he was contributing. He would not let anyone else do "his job." This removed the "us and them" from the equation—we could easily have been them, and fate could have altered their situation and they could have been us.

So why does this happen? Why is one person dealt such a rough deal as they enter life, with some kind of palsy or retardation or autism or other form of challenge? What is mirrored in us by this process? By serving as companions to these dear individuals, we began to recognize and clarify ways in which we were healthy and also unhealthy, not balanced by some extreme part of personality or constitutional makeup, which our charges so aptly shed light on for us. This approach was quite artful in another way, in that it recognized the therapeutic moment. How does something get to a diseased state? What brings it back or moves it through to a healthier balance again?

In every aspect of daily life there were opportunities for healing. With the right awareness, the right intent, small steps could be made that in the long run created changes.

There were so many ways to work on this issue. Is it best achieved through a type of physical movement or artistic expression, or through the use of hydrotherapy, trampoline, or drama? Would massage ease the problem when combined with special oils infused with specific botanicals? Is it something that can be addressed as one works in soil, or with an animal, as in therapeutic riding? Is it something that all those who work with this person should hold in mind, a meditation creating a supportive consciousness?

Because this community was based on Steiner's work, and in this approach there is a belief we have more than one lifetime, some of this work was going to take more than one lifetime to bring to fruition. For example, there was a strongly held belief that it was very important to expose severely handicapped children to as much nature and natural experiences as possible, because this would be internalized by them for their next life: they would use this as the basis for the building blocks of their new body. Whether one believes this or not, it is certainly healthier to allow children to be outside, to feel rain and grass, to eat fresh apples from a tree, than to "warehouse" such individuals because of their handicaps.

In every aspect of daily life there were opportunities for healing. With the right awareness, the right intent, small steps could be made that in the long run created changes. No matter how subtle, these were still important goals. Anthroposophists in healing communities and clinics respect and are open to each other's modalities. If the massage therapist could be helpful or the speech therapist should now take over, there was a congenial working relationship among all the individuals that made this openness possible. The physicians and nurses worked side by side with the teachers and workshop leaders, therapists, and houseparents to find ways to bring more harmony and quality to the life of the person with whom they were working. Underlying this was always the belief that this individual is teaching us far more than we will ever be able to teach them.

As you can imagine, this was a challenging lifestyle. I had 24-hour responsibilities, earned the equivalent of just $50 dollars a month, and in some ways, lived an abnormal

normal in order to give those faced with disabilities a more normal life experience. I met some wonderful individuals and learned many practical skills I had somehow avoided in my suburban upbringing. I interacted with people from different cultures and became a world citizen, traveling and working in other communities abroad.

It grew me up and opened my eyes. In the long run, however, I felt drawn to the world outside this "cloister." I felt I needed to have an education in something specific that I could use if I wanted to return to work at Camphill. If my path sent me farther afield, it would enable me to contribute wherever I was. So after four years in Camphill, I left and went to nursing school. Some Camphill staff come through the training program and choose to stay and become members of the community. Others, like me, still feel connected to this work but have moved into different arenas.

CAMPHILL

Camphill communities are residential "life-sharing" communities and schools for adults and children with developmental disabilities, mental health problems , and other special needs. They provide services and support for work, learning, and daily living. There are currently 119 Camphill communities in 23 countries in Europe, North America, southern Africa, and Asia.

....

Chapter 5

Encountering Chronic Illness

There is a big difference between short-term afflictions and chronic illness. Anyone coping with an illness that has been affecting their life over a long period of time knows this. If you have not experienced this, though, it can be difficult to understand the various layers. In this chapter, I am going to describe three different scenarios where chronic illness created challenges.

MY SISTER'S JOURNEY

I still remember my father's drawing of my younger sister after he returned home from the hospital, which he made in order to let my older sister and me know that she had been born. We were very excited to have a new sister, but we had no idea about the challenges she faced.

She had had a difficult entry into the world. My mother in labor felt she needed a Caesarian section, but unfortunately, her delivery was being handled by an intern who thought all women said that when they were in labor, and not by her own GP, who would have paid attention to my mother's intuition. My sister was born weighing over 10 pounds, with the cord wrapped around her neck. Her face was blue from lack of oxygen, which caused a moment of great concern in the delivery room until, fortunately, my sister pinked up quickly.

After bringing my sister home, my mother felt my sister's cry wasn't right and repeatedly questioned her doctors about it. After much persistence on her part, the doctors diagnosed the baby with low thyroid and prescribed the needed medication at four months of age. She also had some physical challenges, which over time were treated and corrected, and she was late in learning to walk.

My sister has never matched any conventional diagnostic grid. She has tended to surpass any limiting prediction of capabilities and has always ended up achieving whatever has been required of her, and more. When she was a baby, she was highly verbal—her first word (which stunned us all) was "stethoscope." She was already reading by the time she was two. She has a great sense of humor and a savant mind with words. She is an accomplished punster, and sometimes in the rapid wordplay my mind is groaning to understand what we are really saying. I have to plead, Mercy! Mercy!

This dear sister of mine is a very gentle person by nature, and I have been concerned about her from an early age due to her various challenges. She and I have always been very connected, and these early experiences have influenced my career in many ways. For me, the experience of having a special sister like this has served as an example of what it means to be "chronic but improving."

When someone is young and the world is unfolding before them, how they are treated, what they are given to explore, and how they are supported is as crucial to their well-being as what they are fed and how they are schooled. When life is going along as it should we don't think about it much. We know that it is important to expose children to as much learning as possible and that comes in many forms. But when a child is born with unique challenges, it feels like a much scarier, unknown process. That's because there is a great deal of uncertainty about how far this child will go in their development and how this will influence the rest of their life. What opportunities will the child have?

I think a parallel experience for a family with healthy children would be when a family is faced with a teenager who is getting into trouble and losing his or her way somehow. The family has done things a certain way, and it may have worked for other siblings successfully, but somehow for this child it is not working. Thoughtful parents will begin to dissect all the influences. Is it their friends? Is it a lack of discipline? Are they uninvolved? Are they passionate about something that helps steer a clear path? Are they depressed? Are their hormones out of whack? Are they bored? Do they need a non-family member mentor? What subtle but profound event will happen to get this teenager back on track?

This hypervigilance is heightened and becomes the normal experience for families with a developmentally disabled member. The emotional as well as financial and community resources of such a family will directly impact how much progress and unfoldment

---

"One interesting phenomenon is that sometimes, with the right circumstances, what was thought to be a limitation can shift and be less limiting. For example, when I worked with developmentally disabled children, I had a child in my group who was incontinent at night. I worked with her for a year, getting up through the night, and by the end of our time together she was managing to stay dry all night long. She was 13 years old, and her parents had never felt that this was going to be possible for her. Being continent opened up more living situation options for her later. This was another example to me of chronic, yet improving."

— Author

can occur, as they work with the hopes they have for this person as well as understanding the limitations.

In a situation that is slightly "off"—that is, counter to what one would consider "normal"—these elements become crucial. Situations like my sister's, for example, inherently involve certain limiting circumstances that cannot be ignored. The ways in which people have interacted with her over the years have made an enormous impact on her. Some of these situations have been positive and affirming, but some individuals have been cruel and mean, abusive even, bullying her because she is different.

This is painful not only for her but for our whole family, and is a source of ongoing concern. How do we protect her from these ignorant, moment-to-moment reactions of uninvolved people? As a family, we just have to hope that the strong foundation we continue to help her build, and all of her more positive experiences, will provide the best opportunities for her to sense herself and her own potential.

When I was seven, I remember we started having family meetings during which my parents helped guide us on our family situation. My parents spoke about the roles we all had within the family and that we had taken on in this lifetime: Mother, Father, Sister, Daughter, Parents, and Siblings. It was their belief that this combination of individuals was no accident, and that we were meant to be together.

They believed that each of us has a whole spirit, a unique essence, and that we are here on Earth to learn, love, and make a difference. Their idea was that the set of circumstances we find ourselves in helps us stay in alignment with our core desire/mission on a soul level. So, even though my sister has some handicaps in life, she is a whole and healthy spirit, and through these challenges she is learning something she needs to experience. It is our job to help her shine through as much as possible and to never forget what is truly operating here. Because of our roles, we were told that we each have a special duty, from our own orientation, to bring our particular strengths and talents to assist her in her situation.

I felt a peership, an equality in all of our efforts. I was the big sister, and I was going to be the best big sister I could be. I was (from my seven-year-old sense of things) going to be as kind and facilitating as I could be to help her achieve her potential. I felt that there was a rightness to why she was bringing these challenges to each individual in the group. We each were supposed to be experiencing something, too, and learning from it. If we denied it, ignored it, wished it wasn't so, we would miss out on something that had been part of the original intention of us coming together, and that would be a true tragedy. This expectation also created a feeling of deep relaxation and rightness underneath everyday living and all the challenges it brings.

I thought all families had such meetings. Of course, as I grew up, I realized this was not the case, but I am so glad we did and that my sister and all of us felt a sense of blessing in our challenges.

MY MOTHER'S JOURNEY

The second personal experience with chronic illness was with my mother. She was a motivational speaker, a great teacher, counselor, and mentor to many people. She was an extrovert and had directed an amateur theater for a number of years. She was a wonderful storyteller, and could build all the details and deliver the punchlines with great effect.

In a deeper sense, she was a teacher to all who knew her because she kept growing herself. She questioned in fundamental ways the assumptions of societies or cultures and sought to go deeper. She had a series of foot concerns and surgeries and was just on her most recent wheelchair stint at the end of an eight-year process when she suffered a severe stroke. She was 63, and her speech needed work, but thankfully her mind and ability to think and express herself remained intact. Physically, she was paralyzed on the left side.

My father called to let us know, and my older sister flew out immediately. I was running an Alzheimer's unit at the time, and all parties decided it would be better for me to come out when she was starting her rehabilitation process. It was hard to wait to fly back to Pennsylvania. When I arrived, my father dropped me off at the hospital, stating that he was going grocery shopping and would be back in about two hours. It had started snowing, and within a short time the area was hit with one of its worst blizzards in years. My father was unable to get back for three days.

I rushed up to see my mother, and it was so hard. This great force in our lives, this person who felt so in alignment with her purpose—how could this be right? How could this be "how things are supposed to be," and that "all things are right with the universe." It felt so wrong.

We cried a lot. I pulled a pad off a gurney and placed it at the end of her bed at night and slept there. I helped with her care during those three days and also assisted the nursing staff with the other patients because they were short-handed with call-ins due to the storm and were expecting an official hospital inspection any day.

I became aware that the staff did not really know how to work with folks with dementia on the unit. Every shift has its required duties, of course, but the nursing staff was waking up these poor elders in the middle of the night to shower them. This was already a very disorienting environment for cognitively functioning patients, but for the already confused person it made their condition worse. The staff was struggling with challenging behaviors and laughing it off, instead of realizing they were terrorizing their charges.

Over the next two weeks, I spent a lot of time informally talking with them, as I had passed muster and was not viewed as "just" being a family member in their midst. As a result, they were able to change their policy regarding required night shift baths and began intentionally not bathing confused residents in the middle of the night.

Thus began a nine-year odyssey that became my personal experience with a "chronic yet transitioning (from our perspective) declining" situation. This is what I feel most families experience with a loved one with a dementia diagnosis such as Alzheimer's, multi-infarct, or frontal lobe. In my mother's case, she would rise to the challenges of her situation and apply herself to the job of recovering; however, she experienced a series of setbacks during her long illness that led, looking back, to an increasing erosion in her abilities. It felt traumatizing and unfair.

I will keep it short, but she was dropped a couple of times during transfers and sustained serious injuries, one of which caused a deep lethargic somnolent state from a head trauma for a period of months. She developed a heart condition and had a breast cancer discovered and successfully removed. She had a leg amputated. Her mother became ill, so we moved my grandmother into my parents' home and increased the amount of caregiver hours to help care for both of them. She then participated in her own mother's seven-month illness and subsequent death. At some point along the way, my father, who had been trying to cope and manage all this, fell into a serious depression. He had to spend time separating from the whole situation and re-find and redefine himself. Although my mother remained supportive of his needs throughout, it added more dimensions to the emotional challenge of the situation.

Some good things happened along the way. At the five-year mark, my mother was able to give a public lecture to one of her favorite groups, which ran annual conferences nearby. To an audience of 200 or more, she shed light on how this process enabled her to work on a level of things she had previously not been able to access. She called the talk "Preparing For a Peaceful Transition."

It turned out that during the time she had been mostly unavailable to us, she had been revisiting aspects of her life in enhanced detail and working on forgiveness. This took the form of forgiving not only those things that had been done to her, or that she recalled participating in toward others, but also of forgiving very subtle things or situations she had not understood were the threads of cause-and-effect connections, and in a state that was somehow between the mundane here-and-now and the hereafter. In these altered states, she was able to glean insights into the work of the soul.

Severe illness causes us to not be able to attend to the business of our normal lives. Although it looked like my mother was practically comatose, in actuality she was having very vivid preoccupations, and to her, vital resolutions of the very core of her life experiences. Some ancient traditions believe that when our physical being is not able to function in a normal way, we are knocked out of commission on an earthly level so that the spirit can fully engage in some deeper work. Afforded the space and time to do it, this can be a very fruitful time for the spirit. Most of the time, there may not be conscious awareness on a day-to-day level, as my mother was able to experience it, but thankfully, she was also able to come out of that state and share the information with us.

Some ancient traditions believe that when our physical being is not able to function in a normal way, we are knocked out of commission on an earthly level, so that the spirit can fully engage in some deeper work. Afforded the space and time to do it, this can be a very fruitful time for the spirit.

During this time, my younger sister had a chance to become more independent and grow up in some ways "off the radar," because we were all so preoccupied with my mother and grandmother. My father took up watercolor painting and enjoys ever-increasing skill and success with this artistic expression. He also found his internal compass again and continued to be part of everything, which has been and continues to be a blessing. We had caregivers come into our lives who, as a result of being in my mother's presence, felt she changed the way they parented and that their children will grow into better individuals due to her influence. Her example of fortitude, optimism, and an unconditional loving approach to everyone and everything was beyond belief. There was not an ounce of bitterness.

I don't think that I could have managed that. When I consider all that my mother endured, I feel sure that I would have been dead long ago or incredibly angry and bitter. I really struggled with this issue. You live a good life and do good work, so shouldn't the spiritual realm reward you with a long and healthy life? What's the point of doing good stuff if you get blasted, damaged, and annihilated along the way?

I am like Brother Leo from the St. Francis story, trying to decide if inspired, passionate beings are lunatics or saints. If you commit to a few basic principles and live your life accordingly, as avatars do, you will ultimately be subjected to lots of trials because the rest of the world doesn't seem to operate that way. Do you abandon your principles because it is too hard? Or do you hunker down and wait for the next onslaught, affirmed in your belief that not only will you overcome but that surviving takes on a level of thriving that without the experience you would not understand the blissful state you've now ascended to?

MY OWN DARK NIGHT OF THE SOUL

When I was 34, I was diagnosed with type 1 diabetes, which is normally a diagnosis children receive and is therefore also referred to as "juvenile diabetes." As a result, I had my own experience of "chronic and sustained."

I discovered that type 1 diabetes can be caused by a virus. I think many people are aware of the virus that causes strep throat, that it can migrate to another part of the body—the heart, for example, where it creates damage to heart valves. The type of virus I had was not strep but a simple flu virus, but it migrated to my pancreas, the organ that manufactures the hormone insulin, which manages the body's response to blood sugar. In an effort to kill the virus, my body mounted an autoimmune response that killed my insulin-producing cells.

This is a situation that is occurring more frequently, with more folks getting diagnosed with type 1 diabetes up to 40 years of age. People start to see diabetes symptoms about six months after having what they thought was a normal flu. Type 1 is different from type 2 diabetes, or "adult-onset diabetes," which is dramatically increasing and is influenced by genetics, obesity, sedentary lifestyles, and high fat/carbohydrate diets.

Needless to say, the fact that I was diagnosed with type 1 diabetes was a shock! I was thin. I thought I was healthy, eating a wholesome diet, running in local road races, enjoying work aligned with my passions. Now I had a chronic illness—a scary chronic illness.

I had one humorous moment on the Alzheimer's unit the day I received "The Phone Call" giving me my diagnosis. I was crying in my office, trying to absorb the impact of the news and trying to pull myself together, when Doris, one of the elders on the unit, happened upon me.

"Oh dear, what's the matter?" she said in her usual, very loud, very scratchy voice.

I told her.

She replied: "Oh, honey, you don't need to worry. I have that, and look at me—I'm fine. You just have to eat right and exercise. You'll be fine. I have taken good care of myself all my life, and it didn't interfere. I did a good job. Look at me. I'm fine now, and you'll be fine." She patted me on the shoulder and wandered out the door of my office again.

I had to laugh somewhat tragically at this point. Doris had never cared well for herself or her diabetes; it was why she had dementia. She had frequently abused her diet, not regulated her blood sugars, and was found in comas requiring hospitalizations. Her hearing loss, her visual impairments, and mainly her dementia were all related to the fact she had not done a "good job" with her chronic illness. And now she was coping with another one. It was one of those poignant moments.

I was confronted with another situation I could not fix. I am used to throwing my energy at things and making them better. These situations over the last years could not be fixed, no matter what I did or thought or tried to do. This was fundamentally disturbing. It is something everyone with a chronic illness suffers.

It is true that with diabetes it is about living a healthy lifestyle. If it is managed properly, the hope is that one can avoid more serious complications. But there is an element of, "You *must* do such and such." Each day is only as good as you make it, so you have to have structure and regularity. This was threatening and enraging for my free-spirited self. With a chronic problem, you go through the stages of grieving over and over. There might be quicker review of these, but every time a situation arises that is influenced by the illness you still find yourself struggling with those steps again.

Because I have been in alternative or complementary fields of medicine as well as Western allopathic medical settings, and live in Boulder, Colorado, many of my friends or support systems felt free to make suggestions about what would cure me. This was hard because, like it or not, I am faced with one incontrovertible fact: I am not producing insulin, and what I need is insulin. Nothing else is going to fix me—not certain kinds of floral tinctures or homeopathic remedies, not supplements from Brazilian jungles, not avoiding eating fat, and so on.

When I finally got the diagnosis, my physician felt that I had probably had it for a year and that I was still in what they call a "honeymoon"—that is, still producing a small amount of insulin and due to my good diet and exercise habits had avoided hospitalization or some other crisis.

What Western medicine could not do was look at the impact on my whole system of having one part of my body not functioning well. You need insulin to get nutrition into your cells. Basically, the reason they used to call type 1 diabetes "wasting disease" was because people were starving. I had high blood sugar, and sugar draws water, so I always felt thirsty and hungry and was losing weight. But without the insulin "key" to "unlock" my cells, this volume of fluid and nutrients would be voided out of my system.

I went to a doctor of Oriental medicine, and we worked together for about six months to address my diabetes, using a combination of acupuncture, nutritional supplements, and treatments for the byproducts of the stress my body had experienced. This felt very helpful and was reorienting to me personally. I was raised on homeopathy and had rarely taken any Western medications in my life—I wouldn't even swallow an aspirin until I was 28—so I was very upset about having to inject myself with insulin regularly and being dependent on a pharmaceutical. When it comes to long-term illnesses, even though you can't "fix" them, I believe you have to find your way with those things you can still do for yourself that feel right to you. The combination of things required to accomplish this is unique for each person, but it helps you feel you are working with your challenge instead of just feeling challenged by it.

I could hear Dr. Williams's voice: "Why do you think you have this illness?" There were a number of thoughts that came up for me, which I can best illustrate by recounting a simple story.

There was once a man who was very quick thinking, strong willed, and assertive—a classic Type A personality. In many ways his chosen career suited him, but it was hard to know if it was the way he was that created the roles he played, or if the roles he played strengthened the skill set he brought to the role. But it was creating an imbalance, and he was overusing these strengths. He started having headaches—once in a while, at first, then more frequently. He went to his doctor, who prescribed a painkiller for his headaches, and as a result they were manageable. This went on for about a year, then his blood pressure started going up. Again, he went to the doctor and got blood pressure medication, and as a result it was manageable. Then about six months after that he had a heart attack and was laid up in the hospital for a couple of weeks. Every time he tried to work while in the hospital his symptoms would return. It disturbed the nurse so much she made him stop.

Who you are and how you function triggers emotional responses and stress, which in turn influences what manifests as illness. Illness has a path. One definition of pain is an increased awareness in a place or area of which you are not usually conscious. Normally, for example, you take your leg for granted, assuming that it is going to move the way you need it to move; otherwise, you are just going to have somatic (sense) impressions from it, such as how your pant legs feel when you get dressed. This impression quickly recedes until something else provides a new input message, such as when you walk by some bushes and a branch rubs against your leg.

When you have a pain in your leg, your body is trying to get your attention. It might be, "You need to pay more attention and use your peripheral vision and not run into branches," or "You need to stop putting your full wallet in your back pocket, because it's putting pressure on the sciatic nerve. That major nerve doesn't function well when something keeps compressing it." The body sends a pain message, a warning, to avoid further complications. If the sciatic nerve gets damaged it can cause foot drop, weakness, atrophy, and so on, as well as ongoing burning pain. Of course, we would like to avoid all that, but sometimes we don't understand the message or it is a harbinger of something greater to come.

In complementary medicine, different approaches look at the dynamic shift between wellness and illness. At what point do things change? And how can you get patients back to a place that supports their own health?

Here's one line of thought about how this gentleman got into the fix he was in.

The story stated he had a Type A personality, so he gravitated toward a job that emphasized these strengths: a high-paced investment firm. If we are doing something that dominates our time, we need to be conscious of what would balance how we use our natural tendencies.

When he started getting headaches, might he at that point have asked himself, "Why?" rather than just treating them into disappearance or maintenance? This is an emotional question as well. How am I feeling about what I am so busy doing? Am I happy? Stressed? Fulfilled? Challenged? Burdened? Pressed? The solution might have been: "I need to work in a garden on my days off, or take a bike ride three evenings a week to decompress from work and be in my body instead of just my head and will. I need to have downtime to do nothing or take naps on Saturday afternoon. My impulse is to do-do-do, but I think the headaches are trying to tell me I also have to be."

Our man ignored the messages his body was sending him, and did not take into account how his feelings and emotions might be impacting his body. This was a person who was not paying attention to how he was driving himself. He has a medical diagnosis, he's not invincible, his body is trying to send the message "We need some kind of adjustment here," but he is still functioning in the same way. What if these messages are an opportunity not to be so one-sided and to force him to develop other parts of himself? Sometimes, life naturally provides us with those opportunities; sometimes, we have to actively pursue more balance; sometimes, we don't know how to do it and need more instruction.

When illness manifests on a physical level, it is in its most gross form; it's having a real impact. Some healers feel you have to revisit in reverse the path that got you here, so some of the investigation is a review of what happened in order to try to retrace things and get to the healing turning point. Sometimes, you heal on different levels, but the physical impact may stay with you the rest of your life. Sometimes, the realm of miracles is possible because the physical is not as concrete as we typically imagine it to be. In a way, it is as if we are in a play and have roles and props and stories to tell. Surprise endings can occur, the story can take a new direction, but it may also be that we are meant to participate with the props and storyline. It is hard to know, considering our often limited perspective.

In anthroposophical medicine, there is a belief that problems with the blood typically relate to an issue with the sense of self. They refer to this as the Ego but do not mean it in the psychological way so many think of ego, as in "egocentric" or "full of ego"; they mean it more as the "I am-ness," the part of you that has an interchange with higher spiritual realities and directs your life in the here and now.

The anthroposophical approach uses a four-part model: the Ego (spirit, sense of self, use of cognitive forces), the Astral (emotional soul level), the Etheric (life force and area of rhythm in one's life), and the Physical (the vehicle with which you manifest yourself in the world). This approach stipulates that the higher forces, Ego and Astral, work in tandem, and that the lower forces, Etheric and Physical, work in tandem. These forces dip in and out of each other; when a diseased state is present, it disturbs the normal balance of things.

> "The doctor I would want for myself or for anyone else I cared about would be one who understands that disease is more than just a clinical entity; it is an experience and a metaphor, with a message that must be listened to."
>
> — Dr. Bernie Siegel
> author, *Love, Medicine, and Miracles*

Looking at my situation, I had to acknowledge that I had been ignoring myself in a fundamental way when dealing with my work, my life, and my relationships. This tendency shifted in a fundamental way when I was forced to pay attention, moment to moment, to my blood chemistry, stabbing myself routinely to check on my blood sugar levels. I had always thought that I was supposed to put self aside in the service of others, but we need to be present for our individual contribution. It's not supposed to be "this or that" but "this *and* that."

I wish I could have learned this in another way. But I have also been humbled by the whole experience. I am far more compassionate—and I was already a very compassionate person. This somehow drove it deeper, drove it home, in a way I can't even articulate. In essence, it has made me better at what I do, working with individuals who are suffering with dynamics bigger than they can control. It constantly pushes my envelope of being more mindful and self-remembering.

This brings me to the story of *The Velveteen Rabbit: Or How Toys Become Real* by Margery Williams. If you are not familiar with this classic children's story, first published in 1922, please try to read it, especially if you are dealing with chronic illness. There is a moment in the story when the Skin Horse is speaking to Rabbit in the nursery about what it means to become real.

> *"What is Real?" asked the Rabbit one day, when they were lying side by side near the nursery fender, before Nana came to tidy the room. "Does it mean having things that buzz inside you and a stick-out handle?"*
>
> *"Real isn't how you are made" said the Skin Horse. "It's a thing that happens to you. When a child loves you for a long, long time, not just to play with but REALLY loves you, then you become Real."*
>
> *"Does it hurt?" asked the Rabbit.*
>
> *"Sometimes" said the Skin Horse, for he was always truthful. "When you are Real you don't mind being hurt."*
>
> *"Does it happen all at once, like being wound up," he asked, "or bit by bit."*
>
> *"It doesn't happen all at once," said the Skin Horse. "You become. It takes a long time. That's why it doesn't often happen to people who break easily or have sharp edges, or who have to be carefully kept. Generally, by the time you are Real, most of your hair has been loved off and your eyes drop out and you get loose in the joints and are very shabby. But these things don't matter at all because once you are Real you can't be ugly except to people who don't understand."*
>
> *"I suppose you are Real?" said the Rabbit. And then he wished he had not said it for he thought the Skin Horse might be sensitive. But the Skin Horse only smiled.*
>
> *"The Boy's Uncle made me Real," he said "That was a great many years ago, but once you are real you can't become unreal again. It lasts for always."*
>
> — Margery Williams, *The Velveteen Rabbit*

How are the traverses of life making me more real? The things that are hard are sanding my edges. The love I feel for others makes me extend myself, not be neatly kept. And find that I don't break, even if something feels like it comes right to the edge of that.

I have often thought about *The Velveteen Rabbit* as I have worked with difficult situations like dementia and its ongoing, relentless quality. What are we at the end? What are we when ego has been rubbed off, when personality no longer influences the situation, when our memories are not utterable or retrievable? What are we when we can't communicate or do the simplest act independently? Do we cease to exist? Or are we closer to our original state, before we added everything on, layer after layer of human stuff? If we are coming closer to God in a purified state, wrought through hard experiences that force us to return to our essence, should we not suspend our judgment?

"Generally, by the time you are Real,
most of your hair has been loved off
and your eyes drop out and you get
loose in the joints and are very shabby.
But these things don't matter at all
because once you are Real
you can't be ugly except to people
who don't understand."

— Margery Williams,
The Velveteen Rabbit

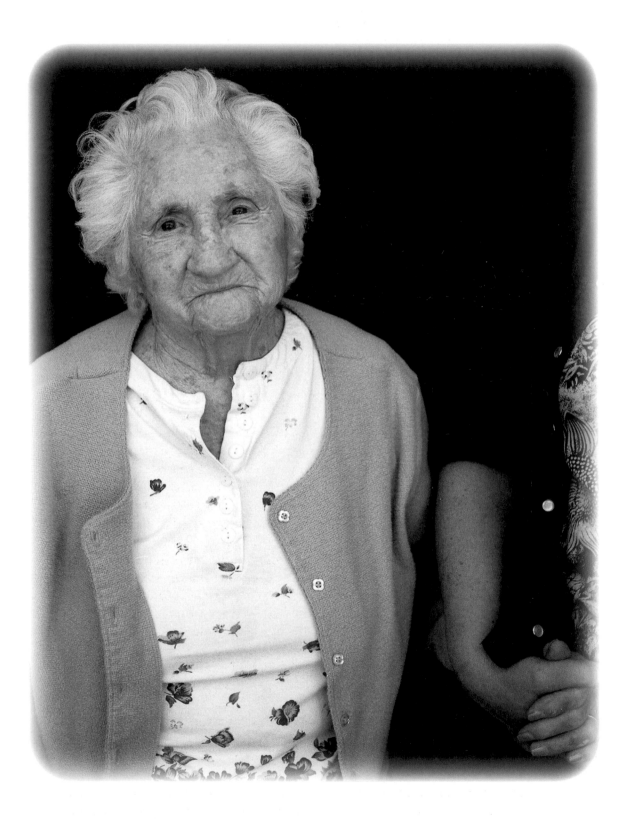

Chapter 6

Dementia as It Relates
to the Elderly

Forty-eight different kinds of dementia have been described. It is challenging to try to gauge what will happen, how it will happen, and when it will happen. Within each dementia diagnosis, there is a unique individual at a certain age, with predispositions and individual resiliency, with greater or lesser resources. Each person has their own individualized emotional makeup, formed through life experiences and the interface with their inner sense of self and purpose and what life has brought them. Some feel they have faced what has confronted them successfully, while others have unresolved issues that still rivet them. Some individuals have put some concerns to rest, feeling they dealt with them appropriately, only to have them resurface through the dementia experience.

Different patterns of decline are associated with each form of dementia, also known as chronic organic brain syndrome. Great strides have been made in understanding the progression of Alzheimer's disease, which makes up more than 50 percent of dementia diagnoses, but I hear the same plea from families when they call wanting a referral for physicians who understand Lewy body, frontal lobe, or Picks dementia. We are pushing the envelope of our knowledge of the disease, and many of these dementias are less known, don't get as much funding or resources, nor receive special attention from general medical practices. This was the case with Alzheimer's disease 20 years ago.

The good news is that many of the advocate and research groups are sharing information. There is a brain consortium on a national level pulling information into one networking source and assisting clinicians, researchers, and educators. Having said this, in a generalized sense we are able to deal with the stages, or phases, folks go through who have a memory loss illness of a chronic sort.

In the early days, we called everything "senility." This meant that through the process of aging, folks began to lose some memory and it was blamed on getting old. We now know that there have to be pathological changes in brain matter and brain chemistry to cause these changes, not specifically age. However, age does have an impact.

The older you are, the more susceptible you are to developing Alzheimer's disease—up to 50 percent of people over the age of 85, according to the latest statistics consulted. Roughly, 5 percent of Alzheimer's diagnoses occur in folks between the ages of 45 and 65 years of age (younger-onset Alzheimer's)—still a low number. But what we experience clinically when we care for folks with younger-onset Alzheimer's is that the disease tends to progress much more quickly: instead of lasting 2–25 years, it is a 2–8-year process.

I have not heard an explanation from researchers, but the first part of my theory is that we don't understand completely how the brain continues to develop through life. In the past, science portrayed the brain as a static, highly functional, underutilized organ. There was a belief that you were born with the amount of brain cells you would have, and you only used a small portion of them. Then greater gains were made studying brains and doing imaging with live subjects, and, in some instances, while doing specific tasks. Neuroscientists began understanding the development of neural pathways and the ever-widening complexity of development through exposure to activities that challenged our growth. Studies done in the past that consisted of depriving babies of stimulus, or observing unfortunate deprivation settings like the orphanages in Romania, showed clear evidence of something every mother or preschool teacher knows: you have to expose developing brains to stimulus and future opportunities for that infant or child to be able to depend on it. More attention has also been paid to the role of growth factors and hormones in influencing brain health. This is one of the main cutting-edge areas of research today.

The older you are, the more susceptible you are to developing Alzheimer's disease—up to 50 percent of people over the age of 85, according to the latest statistics. Roughly, 5 percent of Alzheimer's diagnoses occur in folks between the ages of 45 and 65 years of age.

The famed Nun Study, which author David Snowdon, PhD, describes in his book *Aging with Grace: What The Nun Study Teaches Us About Leading Longer, Healthier, and More Meaningful Lives*, deepened the discussion by introducing the concept of "idea density." All of the participants in the Nun Study agreed to go through a regular battery of tests related to cognitive function as they aged, and to have their brains autopsied at the end of their life. The sisters lived very similar lifestyles in terms of diet, structure of their day, communal and individual pursuits, and parallel work assignments (a scientist's dream). This allowed the study to focus on very specific factors. At one point during his study, Snowdon discovered a valuable addition to his data, something that provided extra insight into aging when analyzed in a particular way.

It transpired that, early on in their lives, the nuns participating in the study had had to write about their lives and what called them to take this devotional path when applying to the orders they eventually joined. The handwriting and words used in these letters revealed how the nuns thought and how their brains worked. Letters that included multiple descriptors, many ideas within a sentence, were considered High Density. An example would be, "I was born as the sun was rising, on a misty morning, into the joyous embrace of the Kenroy family with two awaiting sisters, and parents John and Mary, on June 15th, 1885, in the county of Cork." Letters using simpler, less complicated verbiage and sentence structuring were considered Low Density. An example of this would be, "I was born in County Cork, on the 15th of June, 1885, the third child to John and Mary Kenroy."

As the study proceeded and the sample groups were aging, some of the nuns were not doing so well on these drills. Researchers expected to find advanced disease in their brains, and to find less evidence of disease in the nuns who had done well on the drills prior to passing. But an interesting thing happened. When they got the brain autopsy reports back from the independent labs, the results did not always correlate. Some elders' brains were riddled with advanced Alzheimer's pathology, but in their everyday functioning these same individuals had been doing better than some of their counterparts who showed little evidence of disease in their brains. What did correlate was the way they had used their brains in their lifetime and the idea density concept. This seems to protect individuals by delaying functional changes or softening their impact. This became the buzz of the AD world, and the concept "Use it or lose it" took on a whole new meaning.

So the second part of my theory is that we don't really know which or how many neural pathways continue to develop as we age, or whether if someone has had an extra 20–30 years of life, this gives them more options when one area is damaged, so that another part of the brain can compensate and pick up the task.

We see this in brain injury recovery, such as in stroke rehab or head trauma. The brain is asked to rewire using repetitive exercises and drills. Weight-bearing exercise plays a part in this as well. Often legs mobilize earlier than an affected arm, and therapists will tell you it is because of weight bearing and the stronger signaling this sends to the brain. We also see this phenomenon in early childhood brain injuries, or in instances where parts of the brain have needed to be removed due to tumors or severe seizures. With no left brain, for example, what should have been a left/right brain activity shifts, so that the right hemisphere of the brain alone starts differentiating into left and right functioning portions. This may not be complete, but it does happen far more than physicians ever thought possible. I think this is why younger people progress with dementia more quickly; they don't have the "extra" neural pathways.

Lastly, what is it that gives someone the tenacity to live a long life? Not that anyone expects or wants a debilitating illness, but as folks age and visualize their future, some of them expect at some point they might need some help, or at some point things may not go as smoothly. Even when we make generalizations about older people's inability to adjust, many of them fundamentally do so in some incredible ways. It's that tenacity and will, and their belief in the sun's rising everyday and their expectation to be a part of it.

Psychologically, a younger person has not risen that many days and can feel broadsided in their trajectory. Since they did not "expect" this in the deepest sense, it feels as if their will disengages or can't engage, so instead of a dance with the changes it becomes a cascading waterfall. For a person diagnosed with younger-onset Alzheimer's, it progresses much more quickly through the cognitive and emotional phases and manifests physically very quickly.

Cardiovascular dementia differs from Alzheimer's. It is a form of dementia that involves cerebral damage due to cardiovascular disease, which impacts and causes damage and functional changes and difficulties to the person's brain. This can be small strokes, or TIA's (transient ischemic attacks), caused by blockages or bleeds in the brain. It can be small incidents undetected by the person or family members over time or noticeable with hospitalizations and subsequent rehabilitation care. High blood pressure can cause this type of damage, as well as blocked carotid arteries, which affect the consistency of blood profusion to the brain, decreasing oxygen and nourishment. Some folks have a mixed diagnosis of cardiovascular dementia and Alzheimer's. For simplicity, we will keep our focus on the more common cardiovascular type first.

Cardiovascular dementia differs from Alzheimer's. It is a form of dementia that involves cerebral damage due to cardiovascular disease, which impacts and causes damage and functional changes and difficulties to the person's brain.

What tends to differ with the cardiovascular type of dementia and its progression is that medications are able to arrest some of the ongoing damage in some individuals, enabling a plateau to occur. In others, the damage continues but is more specific and often more subtle. People with this type of dementia tend to become physically more frail over time. Normal aging takes over when it comes to the type of care needed, rather than the overall wafting off of the person's abilities we see with a classic Alzheimer's diagnosis. Persons with a cardiovascular dementia diagnosis tend to keep aspects of their personality throughout their illness and do not lose themselves in the same way that we see with AD. Here is an example illustrating this concept.

BH

BH came to the AD unit suffering from delirium related to a hip fracture and post-hospitalization. She had a history of high blood pressure, which was controlled with medications. She was about 85 years old and had been living on her own in a three-story house with her poodle. Her family was aware that she had not been eating well and noticed some problems with consistent self-care, such as hygiene, changing clothes, doing laundry, and bathing. Her doctor had diagnosed dementia, so the family set up Meals on Wheels and dropped in to check on her. However, they were in a bit of a quandary, because they knew that she needed more assistance yet she kept adamantly refusing assistance. She had run three restaurants and kicked out two husbands, so no one was going to tell her what to do.

BH was a frugal person. She was in the habit of checking up and down stairs to make sure that her blinds were closed, lights turned off, and that the dog was outside or needed to be called to come in. She also enjoyed drinking highballs. In her senior years, this led to problems, as she would make herself a highball, drink it, then forget that she had done so and fix herself another one. One day the inevitable happened: she tripped over her dog and fell, breaking her hip, after one too many drinks.

She initially had to be restrained in a geri chair with a wedge cushion between her legs to keep her hip repair in proper alignment for healing. This terrified her, and she yelled out constantly and could not hold on to the information that she had broken her hip and it was healing—in her mind, this was torture and she was a prisoner. Fortunately, this time passed quickly, and soon she was walking again and participating in the social life on the unit, and the family decided not to have her move back home.

BH transferred all of her previous patterns to the new living setting. She made rounds, closing all the blinds in every bedroom on the unit, unplugged the TV in the den (while folks were watching it!), and at each meal, asked the staff if Meals on Wheels was coming. She always wanted to make sure the "waitstaff" was paid in the dining room, and would ask for a highball and then wink when she got lemonade or some other option and say, "Hey, Hey! This isn't a highball!" She also wanted to know if her poodle was outside. We let her know the dog was living with her sister, and that was acceptable to her.

She could feed herself. She could dress herself if new outfits were laid out and the dirty laundry was removed from her room at night. She could care for her dentures, and became continent of bowel and bladder again once the injury had healed. She could not cook or clean or keep her medications straight on her own, at this point, but she was very observant and would notify staff of things she observed as she walked the halls: "Those two are fighting," or "That person is on the ground," and my personal favorite, "That person is dead down there." They were not dead—just in a very deep sleep.

RR

The other resident who came into the unit at the same time as BH was a woman about 10 years younger, RR, who had been diagnosed with Alzheimer's disease. Like BH, she was also highly ritualized in the way she spent her time and in what riveted her attention. She did not like lint on clothing, smudges on shoes, hair out of place. She had been an immaculate, organized mom and grandma and had run her own beauty shop. Her family had recognized an increasing pattern of forgetfulness and disorganization in her financial matters, and that she was starting to get lost in familiar settings, so they sought medical advice, which resulted in the Alzheimer's diagnosis.

RR was highly mobile when she came to live with us and needed structured activities to help keep her focused and less anxious. She made rounds also, but she liked the blinds opened. Hallelujah! There was light again in our unit. Each time BH would head down the hall and close all the blinds, RR would soon follow and would open them up again. This went on multiple times a day. The beauty of it was that BH never knew it was RR, so no arguments ensued—just over and over, the discovery that something needed to be done about these blinds, with each responding with her preference.

RR's functional level was the same as BH's on admission. She was continent of bowel and bladder, able to dress herself appropriately with fresh clothes laid out, able to do oral care, and brush her hair. She could not cook or clean for herself or manage her medications, and she was also very verbal, conversational, and social, making observations about things and sharing this with staff and other residents.

Over time these similarities lessened, and a marked gap opened up in what each of the two women could manage. Within three years, RR had lost word-finding abilities and struggled to speak and express herself. She could not button, zip, or tie clothing, and needed full assistance with dressing and grooming. She no longer initiated independent activity of any kind and no longer had a purposeful routine of movement around the unit. The blinds had not been opened for about a year at this point. She was incontinent of bowel and bladder and had become resistant to bathing and any assistance with hygiene.

This was very difficult for her family to cope with, as she had always been so fastidious. Within the year, she started falling and no longer walked. She stopped eating independently and needed to be fed. She suffered from repeated bouts of pneumonia, and the unit doctor suspected aspiration problems (not swallowing properly and getting food particles into the lungs). She died as a result of the last bout of pneumonia.

During this time, BH continued to make rounds on the unit but did them less often, with less intensity. She still asked about her highballs, if the staff was paid, and if Meals on Wheels was delivering, but she did so in more hushed tones instead of yelling across the dining room. Over the next eight years, increased frailty related to aging influenced her care needs more than her dementia, which remained very consistent. She was now 93 and had become incontinent—not because she didn't know what the bathroom was for, but because her muscle tone relaxed too much. She walked only the first three rooms of the hall, looking in, not doing anything with the blinds. She was still restless, still in charge, but did not have the energy to push on and returned to her favorite chair observing what was going on around her. Her appetite lessened, but she still fed herself. Her hands could manage the fine motor skills of utensils and glasses, but she had to be encouraged to drink more. Her cardiovascular dementia progressed gently but allowed her to remain mostly herself. She had a narrower band of preoccupations, less ability to handle complexity or multitasking, but still was fundamentally the person her family had always known. She continued to recognize them and speak to them, but more briefly and going over familiar topics.

That is my experience over and over again when it comes to the difference between Alzheimer's disease and common cardiovascular-related dementia. Alzheimer's is relentless in the way aspects of the person's abilities and unique self-expression waft off. The older one is at diagnosis the gentler this is, but it is global (comprehensive) in its losses. Cardiovascular dementia, on the other hand, tends to look like what we used to call "senile dementia." Individuals with this diagnosis benefit from support and structure, and families and caregivers continue to adjust to the person's particular challenges. When trying to assess life expectancy for such individuals, it is better to look at a number of factors, not just the cardiovascular disease, including the speed of disease progression, experiences of blood relatives, and other co-morbidities in the person. These offer better indicators of how things will progress or change for this person, rather than focusing just on the dementia diagnosis.

....

Chapter 7

Advocates For More Humanized Care

"This isn't my home. This doesn't look anything like my home! You're crazy, and I'm leaving!"

Faced with new circumstances, individuals with memory loss cannot integrate the reality of these new settings into their previous frames of reference. Consider the 90-year-old clinging to her house keys who moved to the nursing home after living in the same building for 40 years. From her point of view, how could this be home? What about the elder who had maintained her family home for 20 years after her spouse had passed away. She had her own kitchen, dining and living rooms, bedrooms, a garden outside, but now suddenly finds herself in a setting with long corridors and large, vacuous spaces meant for 30–60 people, with multiple doors and no access to the outside.

Individuals with short-term memory loss often do not recognize that they need help and aren't managing, and any conversations about where they will move to and when this move will take place are not retained. As a result, in new circumstances, they are constantly confronted inwardly by thoughts such as, "This does not makes sense. This cannot be right. I have to get out of here and get back to a place that makes sense." This can be both literal or take the form of wanting to go back 10–20 years in time, to when these issues did not exist.

There is no doubt that people with memory loss have challenged the status quo of care in long-term care settings, actively forcing changes. A physically disabled resident living in a nursing home but with strong cognitive abilities may patiently wish things were different, in regards to their care or the environment or daily routines, but are often too gracious to say anything. A frightened, angry elder who does not understand something and is vigorously conveying it can be a highly motivating force in an open care setting, and this is a contribution that cannot be underscored enough. With elders like this, we have had to find better solutions simply because their moment-to-moment, nonrational approach to life demands it and no rational, logical dismissal is going to assuage the situation.

Changes have included making the environment feel more residential in scale, with living rooms and other gathering areas more like the size you would have at home. It has meant creating a floor plan that makes sense to these types of residents, with bedrooms located away from common areas. Such residences have access to natural light and multiple exits that allow residents to spend time outside in gardens and on walking paths. It has meant creating activities that are meaningful to such elders, so that they are not bored or stewing, and training staff to focus on strengths rather than weaknesses in these populations. In the past, we did not have such residential memory care settings, but slowly, companies specializing in long-term residential care for seniors have been responding and researching better ways to deal with this issue.

Nursing homes were the first to build secure memory care settings. From a demographics point of view, long-term care companies knew this was a growing need and wanted to respond to it. Between 1985 and 1995, leaders in long-term care developed new buildings or revamped older buildings and opened secure memory care units and developed training for staff and criteria for admission and discharges. They changed the physical design of these spaces after researching what worked well and what didn't.

They looked at the needs of different types of elders diagnosed with dementia and recognized an evolving pattern. Many of their current residents were in the early stages of the disease and would be better off in assisted living, as they were highly active and able in many cases to manage aspects of their personal care independently. Assisted living, for the most part, was less regulated, thereby giving operators more freedom to emphasize social models of care and move away from the obstacles often found in medical models of care. As a result, between 1995 and 2005, more long-term care companies and assisted-living providers started expanding into this market. They designed options for the early stages of care and nursing homes focused on caring for elders in the later stages of dementia, at the point they need more physical assistance.

At the same time, elder day care programs that were cropping up around the country and home care companies found that many of their clients needed assistance due to cognitive concerns. This provided additional motivation to address the need for different types of care settings. Today, there are far more options in dementia care, with services provided at different levels of need.

The introduction of more sophisticated ways of caring for elders with memory problems has had a positive ripple effect in the long-term care of elders, in general, especially those who are not cognitively impaired. Those patient, understanding elders—many of whom wished for less institutional thinking—finally find themselves in settings aimed at the individual. Without the push to address the residential needs of elders with irrational behaviors, this would have taken much longer to manifest. Jarring, unsatisfactory experiences forced residential home operators to create less jarring, more satisfactory experiences for residents, and this has been an enormous contribution to changing eldercare as a whole.

STAGES OF ALZHEIMER'S

People with a memory-loss diagnosis such as Alzheimer's go through various stages. In the early stages of the disease, they are very much themselves. They display normal behaviors and functioning but increased difficulty with executive decision making and short-term memory loss. This progresses to difficulties with impulse control, noticeable changes in personality, and the person's longer-term memory is affected.

Folks in the early stages of Alzheimer's tend to function acceptably in their current environment but need more support and monitoring with bill paying, driving, and household duties and repairs. This can be a difficult balance to sustain. Our task is to support independence, being a good friend or loved one in the person's perception but knowing when to jump in with assistance or limit an activity that is no longer in the best interest of or safe for the person with memory loss.

The introduction of more sophisticated ways of caring for elders with memory problems has had a positive ripple effect in the long-term care of elders, in general, especially those who are not cognitively impaired.

When you have memory loss, you can't connect the dots. You remember portions of things, but there are gaps. If you are able to remember that you are forgetting (and this is an important distinction), there will be various reactions. For some individuals this will be maddening, and they will be more irritated and angry. For others, this will make them depressed and apathetic and prematurely withdraw from activities they previously enjoyed because they feel they can't manage it. This may be embarrassing to them, or they just may get into saying no to everything that is not happening right now. They may feel, "It's safer here. I know what is expected of me here, and I don't know what is expected out there." This disease can cause normally social individuals to become reclusive.

Another reaction is paranoia. Imagine yourself losing items, not being able to find a lot of very important, specific things. You may no longer have insight about your memory issue—you forget that you were forgetting. Because your longer-term memory is available, your self-concept from the recent past is still "I am a competent person, able to multitask and keep track of things." Based on your recollections and the sense that things are disappearing, it may feel as though there is a thief in the house, or that people are intentionally doing this. It is much easier to look in the mirror and say, "The world's gone mad" than to look in the mirror and say, "I'm losing my memory."

This is a coping mechanism. Care and support based on kindness do not involve trying to convince or argue with the person to get them to understand that they are the ones losing these things and that they have memory loss; instead, they involve finding ways to help the needed items to stay found, or making duplicates of certain things so that they are easily and repeatedly available, or being self-deprecating about not being able to find things, either, and joking "Aren't we a pair?!"

All these responses are based on where the person is in their journey through this process, how much insight they have, and what is the best way to work with them. As the individual progresses, these adjustments get much bigger and more constant. There are always approaches we can say generally work, but really it's about adjusting the approaches to the individual. In her book *Validation Breakthrough: Simple Techniques for Communicating with People with Alzheimer's and Other Dementias*, author

Naomi Feil says, "We have to cross to their side of the street. We can't expect them to cross to our side."

"It is my experience when speaking with the residents, all of whom have some sort of dementia, to speak with them as I would anyone else with no memory-impaired issues. No baby talk, just normal speech. Diana is one such resident whom I can speak plainly with. She is constantly looking for her parents. At times she is aware that her parents have passed away. And at other times she finds that notion totally incomprehensible. Every day I am at the salon, several times a day, Donna stops by and with a giggle asks if I have seen her folks, and if I did to let them know where to find her. I agree to do that. Progressively, her dementia symptoms have escalated; anxiety levels are higher, especially at the end of the late afternoon before supper. I used to tell her straight out that her folks have passed on. She would realize that she had known that after all, and thank me for being honest with her about their passing. But then immediately would ask if I had seen her folks. Sometimes I can tell her they are gone, other times depending on her anxiety level, I tell her I will tell them where to find her if they came looking for her."

— Cathy Poole, Licensed Cosmetologist

In the early days, when I first started working with this issue, people would not discuss it. The loved one with the Alzheimer's diagnosis would often not be told what they had for fear of breaking their spirit or their will to live. Thankfully, today we have support groups for the caregivers and the person diagnosed. In the early stages of the disease, you are able to have more candid discussions about how the person diagnosed would like things handled when they are no longer able to tell you. With a functional person, in a healthy family dynamic, you can openly discuss the difficult stuff that can cause family members to wrack themselves with guilt later on if these things did not get talked about.

In the early stages, if you have gotten the diagnosis and have the opportunity, it's very important to get your house in order: arrange powers of attorney while capacity is not in question, complete wills, talk about driving, discuss feelings about when to seek more assistance.

There is no question that the caregiver will need more help and assistance. What is in question is what that will look like, how it will feel, and how it will be paid for. What long-term plans for living situations are preferred by the person diagnosed and by their other family members, spouses, and significant others or friends supporting them?

If the diagnosis is disclosed when the person is in the early stages of the disease, you have the opportunity to work together on ways to strategize around memory concerns. This might include leaving notes, maps, instructions, tape recordings, taking pictures of events and appointments, keeping a calendar, and jotting down simple references of what happened that day or what is going to occur.

Experimenting with different types of clocks can be helpful. Some people will find clocks with traditional faces more useful, while others will find that digital clocks are more effective. Families have also used clocks designed for the blind, which announce the hour, to help someone track time more effectively.

Caregivers have to make a conscious effort to soften their re-activity to the rising repetition of questions and certain "agenda behaviors," or routines. We have all experienced making certain plans or having tasks laid out that we are planning to complete. Even the way we get up in the morning and start our day is a type of routine that can be called agenda behavior. If we were employed at the same business for 30 years, how we got ready for work and where we drove and parked became a repeated pattern.

For persons with memory loss, patterns of activity such as "I have to pay this bill," "I need to phone this person," "I have to go to work now," and "I have to get the children" can become predominant focuses. Minds can get into a groove—persons with memory loss are unable to get themselves out of these grooves.

Sometimes, these patterns revolve around lifetime concerns and unresolved issues, or they may involve just simple things that float up into attention. Because of the memory-impaired person's difficulty holding onto new information, it's as if you didn't tell them. In these circumstances, I cope by pretending it's the first time I heard it, practice living in the moment and not doing addition in my mind, and try to be reassuring. If all else fails and we really are in a "dementia vortex," I try to distract the person, change the subject, or divert their attention.

In one family, the father with the dementia diagnosis had been an accountant. It was impossible to get him to stop sending checks over and over to the same vendors. The family went to the bank, which helped them develop two sets of books, complete with a box of fake checks of a different color. They called the vendors letting them know green checks were void and yellow checks written by them were valid. They controlled the mail, and the bank monitored the numbers on the checks so that Dad could happily write all the checks he wanted without draining his accounts.

Today, many more thoughtful books and speakers are available that explain the disease progression and how to focus on positive interactions rather than decline. The focus now is more on helping loved ones to be effective companions to a person throughout the disease process, employing as much dignity and joy as possible.

THE BEST FRIENDS™ APPROACH

Virginia Bell and David Troxel were on opposite coasts of the country, working with their local Alzheimer's associations and active in memory care training and support. They met at conferences and began discussing the approaches that they felt worked the best, especially in day care settings and with care still at home.

The Best Friends™ Approach to Alzheimer's Care, Bell and Troxel's first book, helped articulate what it means to be a savvy

---

Be Proactive and Prepared

"Know where financial records, insurance information, and other important documents are kept. Arrange POA (Power of Attorney) as early as possible!"

— LuAnn, Daughter

"The person with Alzheimer's disease is in a foreign land all the time. He or she experiences culture shock even in his or her backyard."

— Virginia Bell and David Troxel, *The Best Friends™ Approach to Alzheimer's Care* caregiver and focuses on the relationship between the person with memory loss and those that care for him or her. The authors encourage readers to let go of their concern about what stage the person is in. Instead, they suggest thinking of this person as a good friend with a history, unique interests and experiences, strengths, weaknesses, and idiosyncrasies. The goal is to find ways to engage the person with memory loss over time, changing and adjusting to new and different needs, but holding the life story in mind, as well as learning how to be a kind and compassionate companion.

In their book, the authors were able to articulate very clearly what the elements of that should be and how to provide this approach in practical and meaningful ways. *The Best Friends™ Approach* was so successful that some state health departments now expect staff in memory care setting to be trained in it. This led to *The Best Friends™ Approach* training workbooks, activity books, and a book aimed specifically at caregivers: *The Dignified Life: The Best Friends™ Approach to Alzheimer's Care – A Guide for Care Partners.*

We also now have books written by individuals who have dementia, in order to help others understand their experience. Each stage of this illness causes the caregivers to re-adjust to what is changing, and each stage brings new challenges while easing others.

What we know about a dementia process like Alzheimer's is that it revisits in reverse the developmental stages we have traversed throughout our lives. This process is not a dalliance or a cognitive exercise in life review. This form of life review becomes a visceral recapitulation, a reliving, often with intensification of an aspect of self, thoughts, emotions, functions, or physical abilities before letting them go. At times, an aspect of the person that they were not exhibiting in their life seems to appear, or traits the person always had are exaggerated. At times, the manifestations of the disease feel very psychological and existential; at other times, they feel very physical and related to how the brain functions or how it is being damaged. I will go into more depth regarding that in the chapters that follow and will also address how to be able to recognize the differences.

Chapter 8

Recapitulation and Letting Go

After many years of working with hundreds of families, trying to help people understand where they are in the dementia process, I have found a four-stage system to be the most helpful way to explain it: Stage 1 (Early Stage), Stage 2 (Early Mid-Stage), Stage 3 (Late Mid-Stage), Stage 4 (Late Stage), followed by a Terminal Phase. These stages are important to consider at some length, and I will go into them in some detail in Chapter 9.

For now, though, I want to discuss in general terms some of the loosening in self-concept and relationships that happens in Stage 1 (Early Stage) dementia and how it affects both the individual diagnosed with the disease and those around them. The key words that relate to this stage of dementia for me are "impermanence" and "brilliant."

The concept of *impermanence* is clearly visible in Early Stage changes because, in some cases, individuals have been holding a particular pattern of living for not just years but often decades. It is a significant disruption to all levels of our self-assumptions, and although we know impermanence is all around us, Early Stage dementia really heightens the view and steepens the learning curve. Understanding that impermanence is strongly manifesting throughout the stages helps caregivers steady themselves by keeping part of their perspective aware. Things are changing.

Brilliant is not a word one would typically associate with a discussion about dementia. I, however, use this word often to specifically describe moments with individuals with memory loss, and in order to bring awareness to the power of being. There are "brilliant" things being conveyed every day in our interactions with those who are considered "impaired"—gems of sparkling beauty and insights of great wisdom, all spoken in few words from the depths of dementia's altered states. If you stay open, there are great treasures to be found.

Each individual is also like an artist's palette, with hues and shades of what was unique and special to them—something no other person has. We are all part of humanity, but we are each unique in our life experiences and perspectives. As dementia progresses, the palette shifts and changes, highlighting or intensifying those hues or withdrawing and diminishing certain shades and aspects of the individual that defined them or was a subtle part of them.

I have observed these changes and shifts. Modern special effects could try to convey this, with an orchestra playing an incredible piece of music in the background and an enormous sea of color moving in front of us, shifting and changing, based on what is playing and the light reflected on the massive body of water. At first the person is on the shore. Then they become the ocean. And then they are transformed again and found to be in the light. It's hard to describe but palpable when I tune into it. Each painting before the stage description is an attempt to capture some of that, and allow a space to pause and just be, in the process of working to understand more.

Think about your own relationship to change and impermanence in your life. You may find that the stress you are experiencing with the Early Stage dementia diagnosis of a loved one is magnified for you because of your underlying (unconscious) resistance to these changes. You may become aware of your role in the dynamic between your loved one with memory loss and you. Think about what you are bringing to the table that impacts your responses, not just what the person in Early Stage is doing that causes you to react.

This process of self-examination is extremely difficult for most of us, yet it needs to have its voice alongside the grief you are feeling. Becoming more self-aware can help ease some of the stress. It doesn't take away the experience, but it can guide you in finding more support as you identify which aspects of your loved one's dementia diagnosis are the most challenging for you.

Early Stage dementia impacts the areas of function we developed late in life: our executive decision making, judgments and common sense, multitasking, responsibilities such as bill paying, driving, how we have managed a home, social interests, jobs, or retirement lifestyles. This is the outer expression of our sense of self—our ego in its highest functioning aspect. I do not mean ego as in egotistical but in the way we feel ourselves in the world we recognize—our personality and what others interface with when coming in contact with us. Early Stage is the loss of everything we manage as an adult. It is the loss of adult learning.

What I also observe and sense is a rocking and shaking and loosening of that part of us that is our outermost, worldly self. Dementia provides an opportunity to return to essence, and its pathway causes disruption and losses at every level of development in a lifetime. Of course, the health of the ego and the natural vitalities of the individual cause them to rise up and struggle against this.

In Early Stage, one often sees an intensification of moods, behaviors, and attitudes related to a person's sense of "I am in control. I am in charge of my life." This is the initial homeostatic principle of the body at work, trying to adjust and overcome this impending loss. However, if the person is showing significant short-term memory loss and other symptoms, the brain has been on a declining trajectory for some time. It has used its last resources to try to compensate and can't conceal the damage any longer with alternative neural pathways. There will still be "good" (more lucid) and "bad" (more confused) days. However, going back to "normal" is not a possibility.

Early Stage is the loss of everything we manage as an adult. It is the loss of adult learning.

The spirit penetrates the body as a vehicle for its intention in this life. Alzheimer's is an "excarnating," displacing disease to the individual. People with this diagnosis will speak of "gaps." They are flowing fully in a particular activity or having an animated, engaging conversation and all of a sudden it goes "blank." He or she will say, "I can't remember what I was doing or saying. No matter how much I try to bring back whatever it was, it's gone." This is a particularly painful stage for the individual because they are able to observe these changes and lack of ability, or compare themselves to the self of their recent past. They are used to being able to call on their ego to manage their day; suddenly, they still have their day but an inconsistently available ego.

One of the challenges that can occur is excessive rigidity. "No, I won't go to the doctor. No, I won't come and live with you. No, I will not have some stranger coming to my house. I will fire them if you bring someone in!" And so it goes. It is a desperate assertion to maintain everything exactly as it is right now. It is like standing with your feet in the sand in the ocean. Initially, you are stable as the waves come in, but eventually you are not able to stand on this eroding foundation. Without insight into what is changing, what is eroding, your perception tells you to stand your ground. You (the big you) will prevail. It parallels our culture's pervasive denial of death. "If I just live, live, live, and do not acknowledge that death occurs, I won't die, right?" We know this is foolish, yet many of us address our own mortality in this way.

I think of this stage as, in some ways, like closing up permanently a vacation home that has been in the family a long time. How would that make me feel? What would I need to do to savor, honor, reminisce, and organize to get it ready, to get myself ready to let it go? I would roam through it and think about the experiences we had there. I might sit looking at different views and listen to the birds, or the sounds of the lake or woods. I might spring into activity and pack boxes. I might need to sit in every chair. I might find myself having to nap because the whole process was too overwhelming. I might cry. I might find something to be annoyed about because I didn't know I wanted to cry, or because I needed to mobilize myself out of my inertia.

The main idea here is that we are not closing up the home we normally live in; it is (as we used to say in my family) the "plussage," the extraneous enhancements we have made in our lives that are being let go—just as persons with memory loss are losing the aspects of themselves that were the latest and greatest achievements from their lives as a whole. They are not terminal yet, but they are on a terminal path.

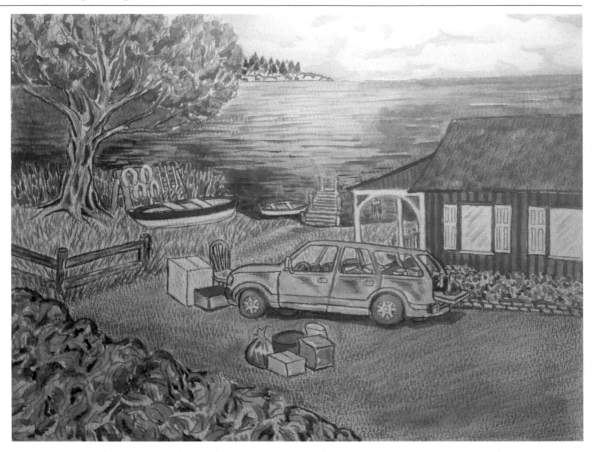

It is difficult and emotional to feel this loss. People with memory loss are still managing many things. They have many strengths, many abilities. There is often a tendency to focus sharply on what is missing, what is lost, rather than on what remains. Sometimes, in our losses, we become more aware of what value those things had for us, making us appreciate more the things we tended to take for granted. In essence, the person is packing up that vacation home, but their everyday self is not aware that this is occurring.

I focus on remaining strengths. I marvel at people's ability to adjust, cope, manage, and make an effort within the context of the changes that are occurring. I feel compassion at the pain they are feeling and the courage the human spirit shows, and wistful about what is disappearing. And it's hard. There is an old verse called "The Weaver's Prayer" that I will find my mind turning to when unable to make sense of things. I also trust that there is some reason for this—some bigger plan I don't have insight into.

My mother said the true definition of "being ordained" is the ability to absorb fear at a threshold. She felt that the role the person takes—whether assisting others with commitment or transitions in this life or out of this life—absorbs some of the fear of that moment for the person and assists them with the leap into what is next. Holding the space, bearing witness, and the religious practice of creating a ritual are all part of the process. She also felt that there are many ordained individuals who are walking about on our planet who don't necessarily wear a clerical collar but function in this way for others around them.

I feel that there are many caregivers, both professional and lay, or family caregivers, who are doing just this every day in their work, absorbing the fear of what is changing and staying by the person's side. The Alzheimer's Association's original tagline, "Someone to stand by you," recognized this, too. The sense of being alone can add such a feeling of desperation to difficult situations. When you share this experience with someone else, it is still hard but it can feel more bearable. The process confirms over and over again that we will endure and find our way through this.

The caregiver, or as we sometimes now say, care partner, is faced with how to work with the person's sense of themselves and the reality of what they are observing day to day. The question is how to approach these issues without over-stepping boundaries and being too invasive or at worst breaking the person's spirit? In spousal relationships, this is particularly devastating because of the partnership role one assumes in this life.

The Weaver's Prayer

My life is but a weaving between my Lord and me
He chooseth all the colors and he weavest steadily
At times he weaves in sorrow and I with foolish pride
Forget he sees the upper and I the underside.

Not till the loom is silent, and the shuttles cease to fly
Shall God unroll the canvas and reveal the reasons why
The dark threads are as needful in the weaver's skillful hands
As the threads of gold and silver in the pattern he has planned.

A couple is usually clear about, "I manage these things, you manage those other things, and you are the person with whom I share my life, my feelings, my hopes, and dreams." Suddenly, one must take on guiding and supporting the other person therapeutically, which changes their relationship.

Some couples have entrenched ways of being together or individual frailties that make it impossible to adjust. An example is the "healthier" person in the couple yelling at the other for not remembering what was just said. Yes, they went to the doctor appointment, too, and got the news that the person really does have a memory problem. But they may have been interacting in this way for 60 years and things may never change. They may be so frightened at the loss in their own life that they can't manage to encompass and support the other person. This fear may manifest as anger and depression, so that in these situations others will need to step in to provide oversight and lighten the load for the partner without the disease.

In some situations, family or other support systems need to step in to protect the caregiver (spouse, child, or other relative) from the wrath or changing behaviors of the person with memory loss, or if the caregiver's treatment of the person with memory loss is abusive and requires intervention. No matter what role this person has previously played in the life of the person diagnosed with dementia, it cannot be a fixed expectation in these circumstances that they will be able to manage their care, either from the start or as the stages progress. If the caregiver thinks they *should* do it, or guilt is the major driver, this will not create sustained loving responses to the changing needs. There has to be an underlying willingness—a really wanting to be there in this role—for there to be a major element of success, in addition to support systems, education, and planned breaks that will sustain the caregiver.

Even though we typically don't view any of this as a blessing, in some families the child of a parent with the disease may find the caregiving dynamic easier to manage. The majority of children separate from their parents and establish living situations and patterns in their lives that are distinct from those of their elders. This means that in times of stress, they are able to withdraw and resource themselves by tapping into a different environment and ambiance. Even though they are coping with the changing needs of their loved one, their normal lives are still ongoing. It helps somewhat with equilibrium and having a refuge for objectivity, but it is no less difficult emotionally when the relationship has been one of evolved peership and friendship.

Another challenge to this process is unfinished business from the memory-impaired person's life that has caused difficult or estranged family dynamics. I overheard one family member say, "Alzheimer's should only happen to the strongest of families." This process will bring things up and challenge everyone, even in the best of circumstances. There may be complicated issues regarding limited resources, either financial or situational or involving supportive social networks.

Many elders have moved during retirement, or children have relocated for their careers, and the diagnosis of dementia and subsequent adjustment may pull the diagnosed family member out of his or her community and cause them to feel displaced on top of dealing with the stresses of the disease. One area may have more resources than another, and this may be a leading consideration in deciding on any changes that need to be made. The sense of what is organic for the individual is no longer part of the equation, so the move has to then be a question of the best timing in terms of the disease and their ability to adjust.

It can also be a time of healing, of resolution, and of experiencing new things in different ways. Focusing on the strengths of the situation or the people involved can sometimes help balance the frustrations and challenges that come up.

What I have observed is that people with memory loss feel that they are losing control, and this is the deeper reality. They may be raging against this shift, and the people they love the most are the ones they can "trust" to be able to handle their expression of their deepest fears. These reactions are not conscious or done intentionally. Sometimes in Early Stage dementia, families are not even aware that there is an impending dementia diagnosis. They view the person's behavior as simply bizarre, manipulative, or a manifestation of a mental health issue, as in depression. It is very difficult to suddenly act and behave differently in response to these anomalies, unless a recognizable pattern starts occurring. Hindsight often causes some caregivers grief and guilt about how they reacted or responded to these early behaviors.

We live so deeply in our assumptions about each other and the roles we play that we may not be aware of them on the conscious level. For example, Dad is Dad, daughter is daughter; each likes or dislikes certain things, and each has habits and easily defined patterns. When suddenly the most loving person you have known in your life is raging, accusing you of having stolen the car or the billfold, this can be a shocking and devastating experience.

In understanding how this feels to the person who is raging, we need to consider how through our things, our belongings, we define ourselves symbolically. Our "stuff" often says a lot about how we are feeling or about how we perceive ourselves at a particular time in our lives. Sometimes, these needs are driven by what we perceive as cultural norms ("If I am in this economic stratum, I should have these particular things"). Our attitudes might be inherited from family members we interacted with in the past. Frugal or extravagant approaches, such as "We might need this for the future" or "That is too fancy for me," are examples. A feeling of deserving or not deserving something can have its origins in the early years of life. By observing how a person relates to their belongings, you can glean information about how they view themselves.

For family members, it is important to forgive yourself for such early missteps and your innocence. You truly did not know what was happening. Waking up can be shocking, like a tornado in a sleepy pastoral scene. When you realize that you are "not in Kansas anymore," you can also start working on finding the tools you need to help you on this journey and remain the trusted loved one you have always been for the person with the disease.

> "Anger, confusion, acceptance, and deep love is the journey that I took in the care of my father, Frolyn. The resentment of having to go through this 'experience,' the frustration of your loved one not being able to shake it off and to fight this 'condition,' the self-pity you may feel that eventually will have no place as the days turn into weeks turn into months. You begin to realize that the aforementioned is nothing compared to the fear and confusion that your loved one feels deep inside, which cannot be expressed but only seen in their eyes.
>
> It was a challenge for me, but my advice to others going through this journey is to get to the acceptance stage sooner rather than later. Decide to let go of the things from your past that you may have carried with you that you now realize are actually very small. Forgive, and ask for forgiveness, and show them love. That can come in sharing of simple stories from the day and from days long since past. It can come in the brushing of their hair, touching of their hand, and even a kiss on the cheek or forehead from a son to a father. They need this comfort and care in this journey, and what you will realize is so do you."
>
> Jeff, Son

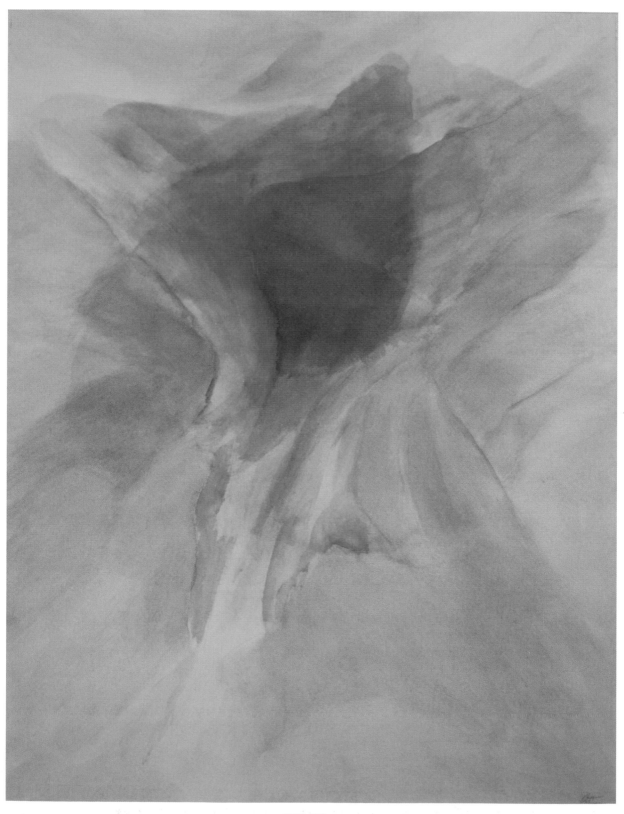

STAGE 1

Chapter 9

Describing the Stages of Dementia

Dementia can be said to fall into four different specific stages, and one final phase. I have called these Stage 1 (Early Stage), Stage 2 (Early Mid-Stage), Stage 3 (Late Mid-Stage), Stage 4 (Late Stage), and Terminal Phase. This chapter looks at the different stages in detail.

STAGE 1
The Loss of Adult Learning
The Realm of Thinking, Memory, and Judgment – Early Stage

Early in Stage 1 dementia, the person with memory loss is struggling with gaps in their awareness and often lacks insight about this issue. Our short-term memory helps us track activities in our schedule, find where we placed items, and absorb what is being discussed in conversations. Taking prescription medicine or bathing in the morning may be an acknowledged part of someone's long-term habits ("Yes, I always bathe every morning") without recognizing that, in fact, this did not happen today.

Driving a vehicle or other executive decision-making skills, such as paying bills and maintaining correspondence, will become increasingly more challenging. Getting lost and missing or repeating payments on bills may cause havoc with personal finances and lead to overall safety concerns. However conscious they may be of it, the person is trying to stay in control and compensate for these challenges.

The dance the caregiver must do is to support this person's independence while trying to assist and safeguard their overall functioning. This may be viewed as interference and cause great stress in the interpersonal dynamics between the caregiver and the person with memory loss. In early stages, we also see social skills and impulse control affected. This may manifest to family members as personality changes, difficulty with mood, depression, apathy, and increased irritability and a lack of "filtering" on comments said to the person closest to the situation. There may not be a diagnosis, or caregivers may still be adjusting to what is new or different in the situation and revert to old habits themselves in dealing with the person with memory loss. This is mentally the most challenging stage.

COMMON BEHAVIORS IN STAGE 1

Repetitive questions, anger and irritation, frustration, loss of confidence, anxiety, over-controlling reactions to certain situations, losing things, blaming, getting lost, not managing to initiate or complete tasks, getting into agenda behaviors or agenda topics and being unable to switch to other things or activities, personal grooming slipping, not eating or drinking regularly, not taking medications appropriately, feeling paranoid and mistrusting, reclusive or not wanting to participate in activities they previously enjoyed, and changes in sleep patterns.

Stage 1 Communication Changes
- Word-finding difficulties and problems with finishing sentences.
- Abstract thinking becomes challenging; more comfort found with concrete ideas.
- Can comprehend most conversations, but not all; has poor recall of content of dialogue shortly after it has occurred.
- Continues to be able to write, but family may notice subtle changes in fluidity of handwriting or the vocabulary used.
- Able to use clocks, watches, and calendars.
- Person demonstrates previous social abilities but hesitates or seeks out others to respond if there is a need for detailed answers. Family members or friends may notice subtle changes with initiative or less breadth of content. Described as "a flattening or narrowing of expression of self."

For the Person with the Diagnosis
- Confide in family or close friends.
- Visit an MD interested in a thorough evaluation and who welcomes a team approach.
- Stress can worsen these symptoms, so look at simplifying life. Structure your day differently, clear and sort clutter, and delegate where you can.
- Join a stage 1 support group.
- Plan for the future and make decisions regarding legal, financial, and medical wishes.
- Discuss at what point driving should be shifted to someone else.
- Express, express, express. Tell the people you love that you love them.
- Because you are aware that you are forgetting, forgive yourself. Ask for help.

For the Caregivers
- Assist the person in getting the right diagnosis.
- Observe the person for depression and try to work toward open expression about the issues and concerns.
- Look at your own issues around memory loss and aging.
- Look at how your role will change regarding this person.
- Help plan and educate yourself about the disease.

- Assist with getting legal, financial, and medical plans in order.
- Help monitor and reinforce driving decisions.

Activities that Assist with this Phase
- Continue activities of interest as much as possible.
- Mobilize social circle to maintain level and discuss where extra support is needed (i.e., shorter time spans).
- Emphasize strengths (i.e., long-term memory, automatic gross motor skills).
- Record stories. Make photo albums. Visit relatives and friends.
- Enjoying doing something together is more important than the outcome. Try to let go of the need for control.

Remember: These are losses of adult learning. It is the disease, not a personal affront. Don't argue. The person's reaction and behaviors arise from fear. They are scared.

Tips for Resilience
- Learn to shrug your shoulders.
- Learn to ask for help.
- Bless what is here now.
- Prepare for what is next.
- Look at change and how you handle it.
- Look at roles. Say what you need to say.
- Have compassion. The person's anguish is greatest in the first stage.

"When my mother was diagnosed with Alzheimer's, we cried together, and she apologized for what I would have to endure. When I lose patience I remember the apology, smile, and forgive. There is a community of residents/visitors/family/friends/caregivers that share the end days of our loved ones. We support each other. I have been given a window into other people's lives.

Family and friends recount the lives of the silent and living:
'We traveled all over the world together.'
'She started a credit union.'
'He was a builder.'
'She was an artist.'
'He was a doctor.'
'She was my professor.'
'She raised six children.'

I have been given a choice. I can hide behind my sadness and loss, or I can make a difference. I can be there. I can be present to my loved one. I can be present to the other residents and speak to them as adults, as real people. Taking care of our aging parents is a spiritual responsibility. What we do teaches the next generation. What we do answers that echoing question, 'Who are you?'"

— B. Valerie Peckler, Daughter

STAGE 2

STAGE 2
The Loss of Adolescent Learning
The Realm of Feelings and Emotions – Early Middle Stage

Stage 2, or Early Middle Stage, dementia involves entering the landscape of emotions. In some ways, this is reminiscent of the uneven feelings of our teenage experience, with changing drives, energy levels, and interests. When I observe teenagers today, I see many commonalities with some of the elders I work with in this stage.

In some individuals, there is a shift from autonomy to relying much more on others, either a particular person or a group for opinions, direction, or friendships. They are revisiting that stage of development, but instead of becoming more certain of themselves, they are signaling more uncertainty. It is as if the crisp edges of the person's defined sense of self are softening and blurring, so that they now have to look to their social milieu for self-definition rather than continuing to sustain their own identity.

Some families report that the person is following them around, or that the caregiver cannot even use the bathroom without the person knocking on the door, trying to get in to see them. In a community setting, they will find a peer and supplant this same behavior they showed with their primary caregiver by following this peer around. It is perfect when both parties want this, but it becomes challenging when one or the other feels hampered, smothered, followed, or harassed.

Tact is a social skill that gets honed in adolescent years but may be dropped in dementia. One elder will scold another because of a perceived social breach, but the person doing the scolding is also being tactless. They have no insight regarding this issue or the ability to stop this impulsive reaction.

Structure becomes very important, especially regarding how the day is scheduled. Channeling energy and engaging different aspects of the person allows the greatest maintenance of strengths; a day that is too loose structurally causes boredom and may lead to unwanted behaviors. This is reminiscent of the way teens can discuss their likes and dislikes, but they are not quite able to structure their days and still need parental oversight to keep things in balance and at their most positive momentum.

A transition occurs during this stage, when family caregivers suddenly become aware that this person no longer understands the broader scope of certain situations. This will affect their ability to drive, and although the person with memory loss may be driving only short distances to still familiar and reliable destinations, their ability to quickly take in an aberrant situation and safely respond to it becomes of great concern. Sometimes, elders will accept a physician's suggestion to stop driving or to retake the driving test

"In the facility where I work two ladies lived together in a companion room. They both had dementia and were not managing well in their homes, so moved to our facility. They became inseparable friends for several years and enjoyed going everywhere together. As their abilities declined, they became increasingly dependent on each other for directions to the bathroom, the dining room, etc. When one of the ladies passed away, the other lady passed not a month later. But their last several years were full of happiness and contentment."

— Judy Dickinson
Concierge and Master Gardener
Program Coordinator

at a state Department of Motor Vehicles office. Occupational therapists often have resources for evaluating this skill set.

Another area of enormous concern is victimization. Unable to use their previous common sense and good judgment, elders may be taken advantage of by unscrupulous strangers or, unfortunately, by family members who fit in this category as well. This can take the form of checks written, accounts cleared out, houses, cars, and other properties signed over without any effort to assure the elder will have some way of managing and have the means to remain self-sufficient financially. I have seen this happen repeatedly over the years, and it is one of the saddest issues I've encountered. It is just too tempting for some people. Honest and caring family members or friends have to put assurances in place and be strategic to sustain resources the elder has worked so hard in his or her own lifetime to develop.

Teens are asking themselves, "Who am I becoming? What am I going to do when I am done with school, when I move out? What am I going to be like when I grow up?" Elders with dementia have the same challenges at this stage, but in reverse. They are asking, "Who have I been? What did I do in my life that I feel good about? What happened in my life that I did not like? How does that make me feel? What is going to happen to me? What has happened to the people I have known and loved? Was I a good parent, a good spouse, a good employee?"

Because long-term memory is more trustworthy and available, their perspective is one that derives from far back in the past. When nothing looks like the landscape they are seeing in their mind, it can be quite jarring at times. They relate to what is around them from the emotions they are feeling rather than from the objective rational parts of themselves they used to consistently employ.

It can be a complex period in the disease. While still able to express themselves, the person may be expunging issues they never voiced or never felt able to deal with. They may be letting such areas see the light of day, as they review their life in the present moment and simultaneously work with the sense impressions that are occurring.

The caregiver may not fully know what the person with memory loss is trying to work through or resolve. However, with an open stance and receptive listening, it can be an opportunity for healing. Even if it is painful, the fact that it has come to the surface and hopefully is dissipating is cause for appreciation. It can give the person a deeper sense of inner peace and be very affirming in the journey you are taking with this loved one. For caregivers working with this stage, a transition is occurring. They may no longer find words and ideas effective to convince the person with memory loss or provide assistance, but they can use their own ability to tap into emotions, and with compassion guide the situation.

As Early Middle stage progresses, we see a continuation of some of the behaviors manifested earlier, but with additional challenges. For some individuals, speech can be affected early in their disease process, while others will remain more verbally fluid late into the disease. If word-finding is impacted, the caregiver will notice initially that finding a word falters, then sentences and "paragraphs" in speech become shortened, and getting across an idea or making a choice become very challenging. The caregiver will need to simplify what he or she is saying and provide word finding (fill in the gaps) to what the person is trying to say to understand the intent. Expressive aphasia is when the person cannot verbally express themselves well; receptive aphasia is when there is difficulty comprehending what is said to them.

There are varying degrees of this, depending on the individual's progression.

An exaggeration of certain aspects of the personality, or heightened activity levels, or what seems to be a total change in personality may take place. This can be challenging to keep up with. Short-term memory loss starts to go farther back in time. In other words, instead of forgetting what happened this morning or last month, the person is unable to recall what happened during the last 5, 10, 20 years. Paradoxically, they are relying on long-term memory more and more, but going farther back in time as the disease progresses.

Expressive aphasia is when the person cannot verbally express themselves well; receptive aphasia is when there is difficulty comprehending what is said to them.

Shared experiences are no longer easily available. The person may not remember this house as the house they have lived in for some time, but feel the house of 30 years ago is where they need to be. They may not remember retiring and feel they should be leaving for work; they may look for "children" that are now grown but feel responsible for their care.

Agenda behaviors can get very complicated, and trying to support the person's perception of things and make the here and now blend with the past can be an exceptional challenge. They may have periods of lucidity and clarity, but these are less frequent while their emotional responses to what is occurring are greater. This is called "incontinence of feelings" in the Validation Therapy approach created by Naomi Feil.

In Early Mid-stage, impulse control is more damaged and the social filters used to screen ourselves are not functioning as well, causing what is on one's mind or the first reaction to something to "pop out." I have also observed that persons with this degree of memory loss are unable to rely on their intellect, so they move from facts into perceptions and feelings in order to navigate their day. The caregiver now must

"Alzheimer's has taught me several things about people in general, and how many outsiders think of them as "less than." It seems as though the public could use a little more education regarding people that have memory loss. I have been amazed to see how our residents come alive and blossom when music is incorporated into their daily lives. Our building is fortunate enough to have ongoing music programs and music therapists that visit weekly, and you can actually see the residents thrive and become more active. We currently have a resident that never danced as a young lady, but once the music starts she begins to dance as though she is lost in time. Even though these dear people have memory loss and are not always able to verbally tell you what their needs are, or what they are thinking, their body movement and facial expression tell the story—a story of a person who is still alive."

— Karrla, Executive Assistant and Lead Concierge

swim in the loved one's realm in order to synchronize. This tends to be the most emotional stage.

COMMON BEHAVIORS FOR THIS PHASE

Problems with judgment and self-neglect are more pronounced in this stage. This often occurs because the person is relying on long-term memory and the habit patterns of many years of life. For example, they may have showered each morning, changed clothes every day, or cared for their dentures at night. Because they cannot remember the short-term memory experience of having done that task this morning or last night, it shifts into assumption, "Of course, I did that. I have always done that." The caregiver knows from looking at the person and their appearance, or having been in the house with them during the last 24 hours that this did not occur.

At times, caregivers will have greater challenges getting certain activities of daily living accomplished. There may be resistance to care and distraction due to agenda behaviors. There is usually a reason, perhaps not rational, that motivates the person with memory loss, and the caregiver has to learn to incorporate it into the tasks at hand.

Caregivers will often see an increase in the following behaviors during this stage: wandering; restlessness; pacing; rummaging and packing; anxiety; frustration; anger; fear; demanding or accusing; resistance; refusals to do certain ADLs, (activities of daily living), such as changing clothes, bathing, brushing teeth, and so on; sundowning (during a particular time of day, most commonly in the afternoon and early evening, there will be an intensification of a person's usual behavior—for example, if they are anxious, they will be much more anxious during that part of the day); overreactions; catastrophic reactions; combativeness; aggressive agitation; calling out; screaming; repeated movements; not recognizing family members in the role they have; clinging to caregivers or firing them; changes in sleep patterns; reversing hours or napping excessively; inappropriate sexual behaviors; incontinence in inappropriate places; layering and/or stripping; delusions; hallucinations; withdrawal or apathy; sensitivities to full moon and weather changes; overstimulation; and illness.

"Agnes had two sons: one who lives in Colorado and one who lives far away in Ohio. She hadn't seen my brother and his wife from Ohio in over a year. The four of us were sitting with Mom in one of the parlors when Agnes began to cry. My wife asked, 'Mom, what's wrong?' Agnes replied, 'My whole family is together again.' We were startled and joyful when at that moment she truly recognized everyone and was happy."

— Ken, Son

Early Stage 2 Communication Changes

- Repetitive concerns or questions, shortened attention span.
- Agenda-driven communication.
- Preservation of some social skills and vague speech (for example, saying something to stay socially engaged without sharing factual information, such as "What did you do today?" "Not much. How about you?" "Do you want apple juice or orange juice?" "Whatever is easiest for you, dear.").
- Need for reorienting information, wayfinding cueing, structure.
- Delusions (having ideas or notions such as "I am still working and must go to work"—they can't remember retiring) and confabulation (not intentional lying—just filling in the conversation with information that may not be true but that surfaces as a response in the brain, such as to the question "What did you do today?," the person responds, "I cooked and worked in the garden," but they have not done either of those activities for the last three years).
- Comprehend most of directed conversation with one other person.
- Some reading intact, but writing becomes impaired and retention may be more of an issue.
- Initiative at times misdirected; inhibition changes.

For the Person with the Diagnosis

- During this phase, the person may forget that they are forgetting and become uneasy at gaps in their memory, demand answers, and begin blaming others. This is a defense mechanism geared toward the survival of the person's sense of self.
- Self-esteem begins to suffer and sense of control is lost, causing depression and anger to arise, with further loss of impulse control. Skeletons come flying out of the closet.
- They need support with maintaining their sense of personal integrity and their need to express themselves.
- They wish to remain in their current setting.

Don't Quit – Just Simplify

"A friend whose mom had been an incredible seamstress before developing Alzheimer's could still be involved in sewing projects. She loved feeling the fabrics and choosing trim. As the disease progressed, she was content with a box of buttons to handle, sort, match, and sort again."

— LuAnn, Daughter

For the Caregivers
- Begin familiarizing yourself with techniques in working with irrational disoriented persons and how to de-escalate situations. Become an expert on "validation" approaches.
- Observe your own body language. Use tone of voice and gestures to assist communication.
- Look at safety issues: driving, stove use, potential wandering.
- Join an Alzheimer's support group, if this hasn't already occurred. Look at ways to maintain living situations: home care, adult day care, case management, respite.
- Have a meeting with friends and family. Educate and openly and lovingly discuss issues and tensions related to the diagnosis. Include them in the process. If religious affiliation is important, include clergy.
- If you have not already done this, please stop using the phrase, "Do you remember?" This is a person with a memory loss diagnosis. That is equivalent to putting someone who uses a wheelchair at the bottom of a mountain and saying, "Go up!" Instead, try using the phrase, "I remember when…" and retelling the story you want to convey without putting the elder on the spot. They can enjoy your story as if it is new, or slowly gain an understanding of what you are speaking about and may be able to enter the conversation with their own recollections.

Music, Music, Music!

"My mom was once a celebrated vocal music teacher and children's choir director. Though her career is long past, music is still a big part of who she is. I play favorite songs on my phone, and we sing. Often, other residents will join us for an impromptu sing-along. When caregivers sing with Mom, she is much more cooperative around activities of daily living. Her physician told me they sang chorus after chorus of 'You are my sunshine' during an exam. The doctor even changed the words to make the physical exam more fun. Instead of 'You are my sunshine,' she sang 'This is your right foot.'"

— LuAnn, Daughter

Activities that Assist with this Phase
- Simplify previous activity and encourage person to do a piece of it instead of the whole thing.
- Channel energy instead of stopping it, i.e., go for long walks and drives, sort papers, cut coupons, shred by hand or by machine, fold laundry, push vacuum, do household chores (rake, sweep, dust, wash windows).

- Make normal routines into a "big deal"—e.g., do a spa day for personal hygiene and ritualize it.
- Look for activities that allow for mutual observation and require less words or cognitive mapping to understand (i.e., Walt Disney film, cartoons, nature hikes, picnics, gardening).
- Order reminiscence materials.

Remember: There are losses of adolescent learning, as well as rising issues around trust, security, safety, and sense of self.

Tips for Resilience
- Anticipate problems. Simplify expectations and environment. Shift to present tense; enjoy the moment.
- Observe for pearls of wisdom.
- Develop listening skills.
- Develop patience and body language skills.
- The need for validation continues to grow. Be creative. Applaud your growing awareness and abilities to care for a person unable to engage with all aspects of our reality.
- Vent to your support systems when you need to.
- Begin focusing on the meaning and practice of "unconditional love."

> "So my favorite memory of Gini was her recalling playing baseball in Nebraska and all the stories (true or not, true to her at the time) whenever I did a range-of-motion exercise with her shoulders. Or whenever I would do tapotement with my fingertips on her back, she'd squeal and tell me how it felt like little bunny rabbits running on her back. Or when I rubbed her back, she'd oooo and aaah and tell me her daddy used to rub her back."
>
> — Amanda McCracken, Massage Therapist

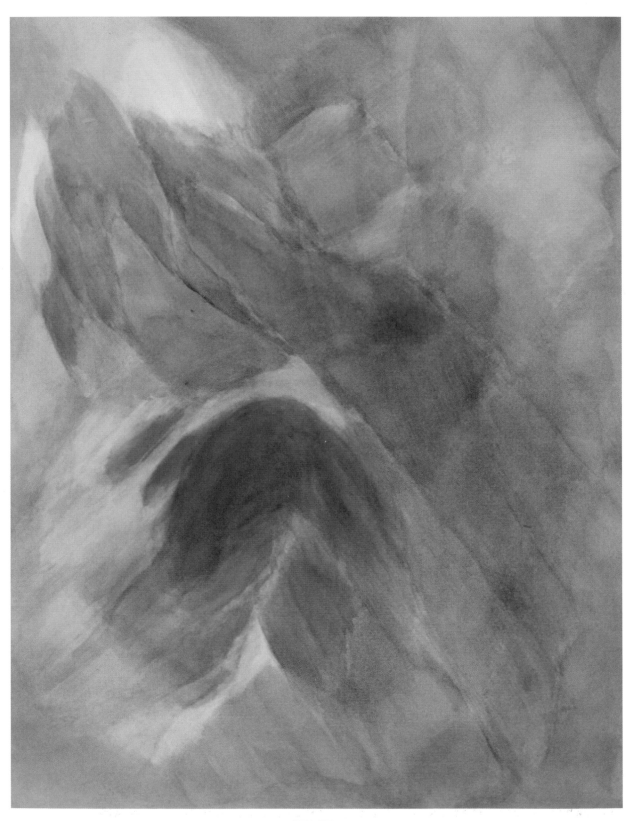

STAGE 3

STAGE 3
The Loss of Childhood Learning
The Realm of Will and How Things Function – Late Middle Stage

The person transitioning to Stage 3, or Late Middle Stage, dementia has had a dementia diagnosis for an extended period of time. The caregivers have made multiple adjustments in their approaches and support. With this shift, we see losses in childhood learning. As children, we learned how things functioned, but in this stage the will to do something is no longer assisted by the memory of how it was done.

The part of the person's brain that initiated a task has been damaged, as well as those parts that helped them navigate each part of the task along the way. Caregivers can help restore the trigger for automatic physical actions by breaking the task into smaller steps and beginning it for the person with memory loss. Using a simple gesture is often more effective than using words, and sometimes is enough to restore the ability to carry out the function; other times, we see the person drift off, unable to sustain the activity.

In childhood, we learn how to dress and button our clothes, how to tie our shoes, how to clean our body as we bathe, how to brush each tooth, how to comb our hair, and how to wash our face. We understand what is needed for follow-up hygiene when we use the restroom. The caregiver is aware that this layer of detail is not occurring and struggles with not being too instructive or pushy while still concerned about how this affects the person's health.

The person no longer asks what time it is, or when something is going to happen. They do not focus on months or years. They have moved completely into the present in their responses. Time appears completely elastic. Everything feels as if it is on its own trajectory, and the caregiver must anticipate how to arrive at appointments on time, and how to keep sleep occurring at night and not too much during the day.

Sensitivity to environmental stimuli increases, so that the full moon and storm fronts bring heightened activity levels. Once the storm arrives, it brings with it increased fatigue and drowsiness. They become much more sensitive to mood, tone of voice, the tempo of what is going on around them. Playing favorite songs and using music in very specific ways can assist caregivers in providing relaxation while providing care. Items such as clothes, teeth, glasses, hearing aids, and other accoutrements become extraneous. They are constantly being fiddled with, removed, hidden, or put in the wrong place. Teeth go in the trash wrapped in tissue or stuffed under a pillow and to the laundry, hearing aids in the denture cup with water. It is frustrating that these tools would help the person understand their world better, but they don't experience it that way; it all feels extraneous.

At the Late Middle Stage, the person with memory loss relates strongly to primal experiences that we all share, such as love of animals, children, music, appreciation for sunshine and its warmth, and companionship with others by sitting close or holding hands. If they sense someone cares for them and allows them to be who they are at this stage, it is recognized and welcomed. This includes the caregiver who can shift to more nonverbal communication and is mindful of how they speak or stand or gesture. They appreciate the person who approaches them and is able to put aside other concerns and be present with them. Memory-loss elders are drawn to such individuals. There may be childlike behavior, but in no way should this person be condescended to or patronized or treated in childish ways. They are always the age they are; they are just relating to things from a much earlier time in their development.

Playing favorite songs and using music in very specific ways can assist caregivers in providing relaxation while providing care.

Visual changes may be more apparent at this stage, caused by damage to the brain and perception not actually from changes in the eyes. Individuals lose peripheral vision as well as depth perception. This is why it is important to approach elders from the front and move into whatever position will help you to be communicating at their eye level. Do this prior to verbally engaging them.

It is helpful throughout the entire progression to explain what is happening, what you are doing, what they might be doing, and who you are in the same way you would with a peer, but perhaps choosing shorter sentences or simpler choices of words at this point. You fill your voice with calm warmth not sticky or sweet language. When the individual with memory loss is surrounded by caregivers who are doing this they are much calmer themselves, have less anxiety, fewer startle responses, and feel safe.

At this stage, heightened vigilance is needed to avoid falls. Elders may not see curb or stair changes, or not comprehend their body needs to do something different to accommodate it, or they may know that they need to but then are unable to get the synapses to fire in order to make their body perform the adjustment. Furniture with arms is helpful to avoid missing chairs and getting in and out of them more easily.

The posture becomes more stooped, and often someone will be seen leaning in one direction or another. Movement patterns can become less diverse and deconditioning cycles begin to occur. At times, private physical therapy sessions with a person who knows how to support functional movement, balance, and strengthening with a client with dementia can help hold this problem at bay (for a time). Walkers can be utilized but for some residents are difficult to accept. If someone feels they are not balanced, and is fearful about falling, the use of a walker is much more acceptable.

If the person has good and bad days and doesn't really sense what the concern is, this will be far more challenging. The use of canes is often questionable because they are used as tools of communication, as in "Get out of my way," "I don't like you," so we often have to remove them. Many of our elders participate in a daily exercise program, and even at this later stage can benefit from this effort. We may see folks participate less consistently or need more individualized instruction and motivation, but when you add up the moments in the session when they were joining in or managing parts of it, it is truly worth encouraging.

At this stage, heightened vigilance is needed to avoid falls.

All of us must really wake up in order to sleep well. We must use energy to have true fatigue. This stage needs support with channeling and expending energy, but it's difficult at times to figure out what one can do with short attention spans and difficulty with performing certain parts of tasks. There are some activities that are possible and in which you will notice a shift to more sensory or nonverbal pursuits, and this will help with preparation for Late Stage dementia.

Incontinence becomes a focus in this stage. Caregivers support the elder with getting to the toilet regularly in order to stay on a pattern that helps reduce accidents and/or wearing sanitary products and still assists the person with a pattern of bathroom visits.

We have elders who are on the move and barely tolerate going in the direction of the bathroom; they want to make one loop in the space and go out again. Caregivers have to be prepared and quick with this type of restless person to avoid frustrating them.

We have elders who are mostly able to use the bathroom independently but at times need assistance with sanitary underwear like Depends. They will just remove the paper underwear when it is soiled and leave it wherever, so then the staff has to figure out who it belongs to and remedy the situation. Our dear Depression-era folks may feel this paper underwear should be rinsed and dried, perhaps placed on lamp shades, which make perfect drying racks for such items. We have elders who have used other options than restrooms in their confused efforts to solve this problem. It makes sense to them in the moment, but in the big scheme of things this is not helpful.

All of these options occur, and it is helpful to talk with other caregivers about strategies if you are having this challenge. Elimination is a very important part of life. As a nurse, I am happy when things are functioning. We want to make sure our elders are not uncomfortable due to elimination problems such as constipation, which can cause combative behaviors, or a urinary tract infection, which can dramatically affect overall abilities as well as put them at risk for sepsis.

This is also an area that affects how we relate to each other. Many family caregivers have felt, at the point of incontinence, that it is really time to get more help. This is especially true if the person with memory loss presents challenging behaviors, or if assisting with this task affects the primary relationship dramatically. There are limits and boundaries to some care situations, and this is one threshold that triggers them.

For perspective, when elders are in this phase, it is helpful to have more things going on around them that are naturally distracting and occupy their interest from moment to moment. This is the advantage of a social setting.

I think every family's goal is to keep the elder integrated in the family and in their home, receiving whatever increased care they need. For some families, this is especially possible if the home is busy with intergenerational activity, pets, or a garden that allow the person with memory loss choices of engagement. It allows that front porch experience of being able to passively observe many things without being asked to actively participate.

Sometimes, the quiet singular focus of a home setting does not provide this. Families report the person sleeping too much, seeming bored, and "getting into trouble." This is another parallel to early childhood. One tended not to put a child on the spot and ask them how they feel, what they are doing, or what they are going to do with their life. One expected children in the flow of things to be gathering experiences—participating at their level while we provide the structure for their growth and experiences without too much insistence on immediate outcomes or productivity.

Elders in this phase have the same need to flow with things in a way that is less riveting. It is relaxing to them to be able to observe and participate in ways that are comfortable to them. Some elders come to memory care settings in the Middle phases because socializing and having peers is important throughout a lifetime.

When a confused elder is interacting constantly with oriented friends and families, it can feel luxurious; everyone is probably compensating for the person's deficits. But there can be times when something is missing. We have elders who befriend each other and have a sense of connection because other people with dementia often do "understand" at a level we can't. It is still important to have oriented folks around to help guide situations when increased confusion coupled with impulse control problems flare. In most cases, though, there is a sense of community that forms when elders with memory loss have opportunities to spend time together in environments that support this natural and important social aspect of life.

The generations who have aged in this most recent era were schooled with memorization as part of their education. There are many elders who are able to recite certain famous speeches or writings with ease, can sing every word of a song, although other word-finding is challenged. They are still harvesting those long-term memories from early in their life, and it gives the person a chance to not feel memory impaired as they recite. I worry about my generation, as this was not part of our education and we won't have these skills to draw on. When the elder speaks of going home, or of wanting certain family members—siblings or parents—it is often the childhood home, with family at the age they were when the person with memory loss was a child.

"Ellen is a resident whose dementia has affected her physically. Her back bends a good 90 degrees, where once she stood as a graceful, slender, tall, six-foot woman. She is a paradox. Her mind is brilliant, yet confusion leads her to remove her clothing. She prefers bare feet. How does she slip out of her one-piece-zipped-to-the-back-of-her-neck outfit without unzipping?! She has been called a Houdini. She loves to crawl on the floor—ever the geologist, her profession, looking for "specimens." She will speak in French, then in Spanish, then back to English. Ellen gives her geology speeches to anyone who is listening. To her, we are her students at the college where she taught in Colorado.

Ellen is a delight to speak with. Some moments seem nonsensical. But mostly, she shares pithy thoughts, if you listen carefully. She even tracks current situations. Once, while sitting in the salon waiting for her hair to be cut, I brought up the name of the actress Gwyneth Paltrow and her mother. I could not remember Gwyneth's mother's name. I said, 'I can see her face and even see the letters of her mother's name, but I cannot remember it.' Without missing a beat, Ellen instantly and without hesitation, said, 'Blythe Danner.' My jaw dropped. I said, 'Ellen you are absolutely correct!' That so impressed me.

The other day, during morning exercise, Gail, the activity leader for that day, asked the group of residents for the name of the actress who at one time was married to Humphrey Bogart. She said that this actress had left a great legacy of films during her lifetime, and that she had suddenly passed away. Ellen once again and without hesitation said, 'Lauren Bacall.' I was working in the salon next to the area where morning exercise was being conducted and could hear the conversation. I just smiled. That Ellen, she is something!"

— Cathy Poole, Licensed Cosmetologist

With recapitulation and life review, the Late Middle stage is about letting go of childhood learning, revisiting how something worked in the process of its undoing, and dealing with the challenge of letting go of these very fundamental abilities. We feel the level of these losses profoundly and act as companions to the individual, finding simpler means to stay connected. We desperately want to retain the previous level of complexity in the expression of this person's broader self. It is important to remember that the traditional and known routes to bridge communication between us are no longer available to them. They have shifted, turning in a direction that we cannot follow. It is important to remember the wholeness of their spirit remains intact. If we stay open, they will find ways to let us know this.

COMMON BEHAVIORS FOR THIS PHASE

When memory loss has progressed to this level, we begin seeing impairments in functioning, with less ability to recognize objects and what to do with them. This is called agnosia, and includes how to dress and in what order, where the toilet is, how to use it, and how to do hygiene tasks in a complete and thorough way. Eating may be done on the move because of increased restlessness. Utensil use may become challenging. Fine motor skills begin to be lost, with gross motor skills remaining. For example, walking is fine but buttoning a shirt is not.

The behaviors mentioned in earlier sections may still be occurring but less intensely around ideas or cognitive preoccupations of early phases. The behaviors tend to be more around moods and movement. This includes greater restlessness, or labile moods; impulsivity that tends to be physically acted out and seems nonsensical, such as taking all the covers off the furniture cushions, removing all clothes out of closets, constantly moving items and hiding them, but not doing this with thoughtfulness about where they are hiding things, physically just moving something from here to there, and in doing so stashing it under or in something. Some earlier behaviors may have lessened or disappeared; others may have intensified.

The reality of any phase in this disease is "This too will pass." So something that can be very challenging and upsetting for a period of time will begin to change, soften, or disappear as the person continues to decline. Another behavior may take its place as the challenging focus, but this, too, will change, soften, or disappear. It's important to be able to see this, because it can help you remain somewhat objective by recognizing the pattern of it all.

The depth of the person's confusion can be quite great at this point, and there may be anxiety, agitation, and aggression toward the caregiver when they are trying to accomplish a task. This reaction is based on a fight-or-flight reaction in the brain and the inability to process what is happening. Calm, slow, paced approaches are needed to de-escalate

Pare It Down

"My mom loved word games like crossword puzzles and Scrabble. A few years ago, she beat nearly every opponent at the game of Scrabble. Even with Alzheimer's, we played almost daily. As that became difficult, I just put the letter tiles out and let her make words. Nowadays, she can't identify a piece of furniture as a chair, but if I ask her to spell the word chair, she says, 'c - h - a - i - r' with no hesitation. We can still enjoy word games!"

— LuAnn, Daughter

this type of response. At times, for safety reasons, medications may need to be used to help the person feel calmer during intimate care. This is the stage of losing how the things basic to our self-care function.

Listen With Your Heart

"My mom still chatters on and on, but very little of what she says makes sense. It would be easy to ignore her talking but I might miss out. One day I told her it was nice to see her. She smiled and said, 'I'm here to satisfy your satisfaction.' How sweet is that?!"

— LuAnn, Daughter

Late Stage 3 Communication Changes
- Word soup, word salad.
- Further loss of impulse control and emotional incontinence.
- Short attention span.
- Repetitive motion, restlessness.
- Ability to tap into long-term memory with songs and school learning.
- Ability to respond to Yes and No questions, echolalia (repeating back what is said to them), aphasia (both receptive and expressive difficulty in understanding what is said to them and difficulty expressing themselves to others due to a loss of word finding).
- Visual changes that affect startle response.
- Use of gestures increases ability to comprehend meaning of interactions.
- Some reading skills remain, but with a greater lack of retention and comprehension decreases.
- Sensitivity to environment, e.g., storm fronts, full moon.
- Short-term illnesses profoundly affect baseline level of abilities. If ill, often communication skills decline during the period of illness.
- Takes less initiative.

For the Person with the Diagnosis

- Need to have lots of space to roam and pace, regular walks, ability to be outside frequently.
- Environment needs to be greatly simplified. Reduce or get rid of TV.
- Stress-related illnesses tend to disappear, and some comfort often increases in the person due to flowing more with the present moment.
- Person starts declassifying their speech and makes free associations at times that are clearer than undiagnosed people's way of speaking.
- They are who they are. Pretenses drop. May need to resolve old issues and experiences in life, but have challenges due to emerging deficits.
- At times, who we are now is more important than who we have been to each other.
- There can be continued incontinence of feeling (Naomi Feil).

For the Caregivers

- Functioning as historian, one can weave through speech difficulties and pick up the essence of what the person is concerned about or trying to say.
- With the help of the MD, review issues, concerns, and medication that can be reduced or discontinued. Ask about the "rule of 6 or less medications" that is recommended, if possible, for individuals over the age of 65. Please see the appendix for recommendations regarding cognitive and behavioral medications.
- Look at wardrobe to see if simplification can be made while still allowing their individuality.
- Increase rhythms in the day, i.e., at regular intervals and times, activity versus resting, outside or inside, and so on. Routines are very important because it allows the person to relax, then be able to draw on extra energies for concentration when needed.
- Allow enough time for activities that cause stress, such as bathing (right time of day, right person, right approach, and so forth). Discuss problem behaviors with others, such as Alzheimer's Disease association, other caregivers, or professional care providers.
- Expect to have more difficulty following the person "in." Unexpressed feelings gain strength and distortion. Expressed feelings lose their strength and leave the person feeling light and healthier. Use this intensity of feeling to clean house, get help, express, and don't bottle up.

Activities that Assist with this Phase
- Encourage whatever piece of the task they can do or try.
- Use "Thank you" instead of "No."
- Increase use of music and visits with animals and children.
- Label all photo albums and pictures in the house.
- Simplify the environment further.
- Enjoy quiet relaxing activities, such as puzzles, looking at picture books or magazines, playing picture bingo, dominos, checkers, preparing green beans, peeling potatoes, or shucking corn. Make drop cookies, cut biscuit dough, read aloud or recite favorite poems, faith-based writings, and other meaningful writings.
- Provide sensory stimulation. Get fresh air and go for regular walks. Sit in the sun, using glider rockers and porch swings. Smell and touch flowers and plant window boxes. Carry or move things. Sit in lawn chairs. Dangle your feet in a wading pool on a hot day.
- Use aromatherapy, textures, and colors of food to enhance sensory experiences.
- Order things like *Reminisce* or *Good Old Days* magazine or activity books such as Minds Alert, which has cognitive stimulation activities such as "A stitch in time saves _____."
- Retell the person's life to them.

Remember: This stage involves the loss of childhood learning. The body instinctually tries to get moving to keep the cognitive wheels turning. Normal behavior can become exaggerated or expressed inappropriately. Try to channel them, instead of stopping them. Disorientation can cause fight-or-flight reactions; work toward de-escalation.

Unfiltered!

"Many people with dementia often lose their 'filters' and say anything and everything. They're as pure and honest as little children. Wouldn't it be nice to just say what you feel once in a while?"

— LuAnn, Daughter

Tips for Resilience

- Humor is an incredible salve.
- Complaining or blaming is often a projection—the person is actually talking about themselves or someone else in their life. Learn not to take it personally.
- Look forward to lucid moments, savor them while they are there, enthusiastically take the pearls that are being dropped.
- Slow down, enjoy the senses. See, hear, taste, smell, and touch the life around you.
- Know that the anguish has, for the most part, lifted from the diagnosed person— they are busy being.
- Focus on companionship. Do things together that don't focus too much on words.
- Your ability to be patient, to anticipate, to be a keen observer will help you in other areas of your life. Share the strength you are developing with others.
- Unconditional love is an exercised skill now.

"I was always amazed by how my very presence would bring out Mom's love. Even when she could not remember my name, she would see me and say things like 'You are so attractive to me!' or 'I love you!' emphatically. It was testament to the energetic connection we had, even when language was eluding her.

One time, she asked me 'Why do you look so nice?' I said, 'Because you love me,' to which she nodded in agreement. Over time, Mom was able more and more to just rest in the undeniable feeling of love she had for me. It made both of us very happy."

— Celeste Niehaus, Daughter

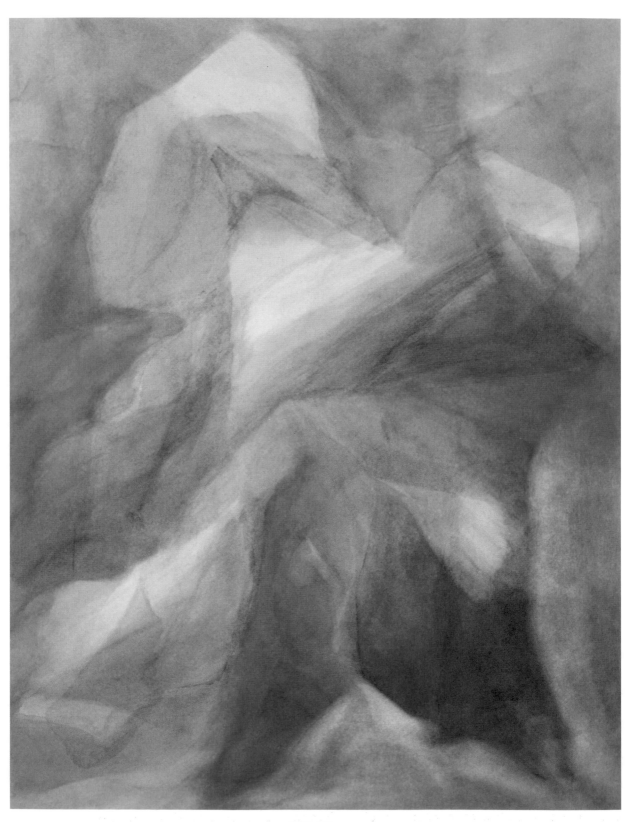

STAGE 4

STAGE 4
The Loss of Infant Learning
The Realm of the Physical Body – Late Stage

In Stage 4, or Late Stage dementia, the caregivers and the person with memory loss have traveled a long way together. If it has not already occurred, the shift involves looking at care decisions based on comfort and quality of life, and not as much on curative approaches. In this stage, elders may spit out medications, even if crushed or in a liquid form. Certain medications don't make sense anymore, such as cholesterol prevention drugs, or an osteoporotic drug that takes years to build bone in the body. Suspected cancers or other illnesses may not be treated when what would have to occur versus the real benefit for the person is weighed. This stage involves the loss of infant learning.

As babies newly arrived on this planet we are like magnets, stuck flat by gravity against whatever surface we are on. Strange things are orbiting around us, which slowly we realize are connected to us. As our bodies start to come under our control we move toward objects, grabbing them with our whole hand in what is called a "palmer grasp" and then, as our grasp becomes more refined, we reach out with individual fingers and hold on to objects in what is called a "pincer grasp." We are frequently tired and need to sleep 18–20 hours, initially.

Our disproportionately large head rolls around on our necks. Our malleable, floppy body finally masters how to stabilize and hold an upright position. Once this strength has developed, we pull our bodies up and, holding on to objects, slowly learn to stand, then walk, then balance with hands free, and finally running.

We learn where nourishment comes from and who brings it, who responds to our needs and how this occurs. We observe, smile, laugh, cry, and make sounds. Slowly, the focus of our sounds begins to imitate the sounds of the words around us. We begin cataloguing what things are called and fold these new words into rudimentary speech, progressing from single words, to sentences, to phrases. We can recognize familiar people, and go through stages of welcoming anyone who interacts with us, to feeling put out by not being around our preferred person. We express ourselves freely and slowly learn about patience, delayed gratification, and controlling our bodily functions.

We want to do things for ourselves—eating, drinking, walking in a certain direction. We find out about the word "No," and we like using that word, eventually we will get fascinated with "Why?" and use it a lot, too. The world is fresh. It is our beginning, and we are laying down the foundations for our participation in the human community. These are all needed steps, and our energy is consumed with the tasks of growing physically, mentally, and emotionally, fueled by spirit longing to do so.

In Late Stage dementia, we are still revisiting in reverse what we developed in this early life stage and letting go of these skills. We lose fine motor skills first, then gross motor skills. Family will notice increased difficulties with buttoning or using utensils at meals. They may have switched already to foods that can be picked up by hand, and now find the person struggling with this and needing to be fed.

The pace of mobility has greatly slowed. Long ago, the person with memory loss knew how to walk briskly, run, and readily adjust their balance if needed. They lost these abilities and their gait shortens to a shuffle and falters. They can't make adjustments for curbs or stairs; even area rugs cause falls. Soon, standing up becomes a challenge, and being able to balance standing and initiating a step is no longer possible.

Family will assist by giving the person a hand, but find, after multiple verbal cues and leaning in to lift, the person is unable to respond and has no way of instructing their body to support the activity being asked of them. Eventually, the person with memory loss will not be able to sit up independently, roll over, or even lift an arm to put it into a sleeve.

In Late Stage dementia, we are still revisiting in reverse what we developed in this early life stage and letting go of these skills. We lose fine motor skills first, then gross motor skills.

Tasks become very physical. What upset the person emotionally in the past will recede and no longer be a preoccupation for the caregiver to focus on. Psychosocial approaches are now eclipsed by highly physical care. There may still be reactivity and resistance that continues to bring an element of struggle into care, but it is driven by not understanding what is happening, and why it is happening. The person is so focused in the moment, with no relationship to what just was, or what will be, that there is little to draw on about why something is a good idea.

We know it is not good to be wet from incontinence, but the person just feels suddenly that their clothes are being removed. We know it is good to drink liquids, but the person feels the glass at their lips and suddenly liquid hitting their lips, as if it were coming out of nowhere. If they feel their thirst they will accept this, but if they do not have that sensation any longer, this will be experienced as strange and that it needs to stop.

One notices the effects of damage to the brain most profoundly at this point. There has been damage all along the way causing the changes, but earlier in the progression, the person's ability to compensate at times and still have moments that connect hides what is transpiring in their brain. We spoke earlier of the process of harvesting emotions and resolving some life experiences as a driver of some of the person's behavior; now, caregivers notice differences in behavior. There is an inability to engage and a clear physical sense to the movement, expressions, and use of sound. Now, the behavior is driven by the brain's ability or inability to process and function in relationship to immediate stimulus.

This stage is an area where I feel we need to do a better job. We have managed to understand and provide improved strategies of care for Early, Middle, and Late Middle stages, but this Late Stage carries some unique challenges, which could be addressed in better ways. It may be that a person can fit into standard skilled care settings at this point because of lack of mobility and total assistance needed with tasks of daily living. Many facilities do not, however, continue a memory care focus, even though this is still the driving factor in changes of ability in the elder. If the staff can be trained in best practices for dementia care, and continue to use these approaches with those residents who need it within their assigned group, it can help this issue. A better solution is to dedicate a portion of the facility to skilled memory care needs and adjust activities and routines to this Late Stage.

To accomplish this, the environment should be smaller and more intimate. The common areas should still be residential in scale, with familiar furnishings and access to the outdoors. There need to be spaces where folks can come together as a group, and areas that can be solitary or host smaller gatherings.

Meals tend to take a long time, so staff need to find ways to lift the mood and still create a dining experience. This means including residents, giving them eye contact, and talking to them without expectation of response but still giving a resident time, just in case they might respond, and helping them not feel rushed or passed over.

It means noticing how we assist them, how noisy we are, how we lift the food or fluid to their mouth. How do we observe their body language and facial expression to assess their connection to us and the task at hand? This is the opportunity for wonderful sensory experiences, providing exquisite touch with basic care, utilizing massage if offered and accepted, range of motion exercises done with music and rhythm, animals and children visiting and being allowed to do their thing in and around the elders.

Consider using aromatherapy in various ways and cooking certain items nearby to allow the body to adjust and anticipate, such as the smell of coffee brewing in the morning. There are so many ways that we can still share the best of our human experience and bring these moments of simple pleasures to them. Other examples are sitting in the sun, feeling a light breeze, being still but being greeted as still present.

I don't feel the elders themselves feel time in the same way at this stage. We may be aware of each passing minute, week, and month, but my sense when I work with elders in this stage is that there is drift or dreamlike feeling to their waking and sleep life. I know when I have been tired and ease into an unexpected nap, I will either be shocked that as long as an hour has passed or only 10 minutes. It feels completely relative—I can never predict whether I think the nap was too long or too short.

Even when we have a good sense of time and its passage, there are moments in all of our experiences when we are not perceiving the passage of time accurately. Looked at from the outside, it may seem to us that at this Late Stage there is great suffering in the endless waiting and stillness the person "endures" in relation to the passage of time. A different way to look at this is to consider the immediate experience the person is having.

When a baby arrives, there is often a lot of joy about this being's arrival. We make the room ready, and try to make sure that everything this new participant in our human community comes into contact with is the best it can be. Things are soft and pretty. We know there needs to be rest and help, and that it will be challenging at times, but we also have excitement about this new life and its future.

I wish we could hold that same stance with Late Stage dementia. The person is preparing to make their transition, they are needing the same kind of help, and we can be celebrating the long and amazing life they did have, and in our care be honoring of that in fundamental ways. Are the baths like spa experiences? The

"Sense of time relaxes. Far less urgency to get somewhere else. There may be thoughts and comments about deceased people as if they're still in this person's active life, and in a way, they are. Another reminder to not judge such a remark because I would say we don't really know. It's a mystery we can recognize and appreciate and be curious about—maybe we don't actually know as much about other realms as we think we do!"

— Ellen
  Geriatric Case Manager

linens soft and lovely? The clothes cozy and comforting? Is there a kind of joy in the air, instead of pity about the journey winding down?

The person is wrapping up the last loose ends and will be transitioning soon. What do we want to share, to tell, to forgive, to ask to be forgiven for, speaking to the whole spirit of the person rather than only the physical aspect in front of us? Many people on this dementia journey have in some ways already "departed" prior to this stage. When someone is participating in the whole extended journey, I tend to ask if this person is still here, what are they working on, and/or who needs them to still be here? How can we support them in a way that is loving and mindful and not harassing and jarring? How can we help those in connection to also prepare to let them go?

Things begin to slow down in Late Stage 4, and the most marked changes are now on a physical level of functioning. The person with memory loss begins having difficulties with walking, using a shuffling gait or stutter step. He or she will be unable to maintain balance and independently transfer or move between sitting and standing and other activities, which leads to immobility and a need for assistance with repositioning and any movement. For example, apraxia causes an inability to self-direct the movements of one's limbs. Moving an arm into a shirt may have a stiff unbending quality, or reaching for a cup causes it to be knocked over.

Things now begin to transition, from the person having some ability to still do some tasks related to dressing, grooming, and bathing to needing help with all these tasks. In the early stages, the caregiver's role is to observe and assist in inconspicuous ways. It grows to include more supervision and active assistance. Finally, it involves giving total assistance with every aspect of daily life.

"I am thinking about Carol. Her neck was perpetually tipped forward. She was constantly in pain, and her mood reflected that. She was crabby and rarely spoke without yelling. Her aides and family tried to get her to wear a neck brace while she was in her wheelchair, but she would tear it off and throw it down. They asked me to massage her to give her strained neck muscles some relief. It didn't go well for our first few visits. She didn't want to be touched. But after some time, she allowed me to be there. It took six weeks—twice a week for a half hour each—to get to the point where I could recline her in her chair and stretch out her neck muscles. I would prop her up with pillows as a sort of support scaffolding and, more than once, she fell asleep there.

Once, I showed up to find her like that, in her chair, with her neck tilted back in a reclining position. But she was all by herself. I never found out who put her there like that.

'Carolyn! I can see your eyes! I'm so lucky!' I said.

She reached out towards my face and said, 'I'm the lucky one.'

I sat in my car after that session and cried. She really touched me."

— Heather, Massage Therapist

"Mom had a wonderful sense of humor, and her wealth of jokes, sarcasm, and expressions were well known to us as we grew up. As the disease progressed, her willingness to cooperate with the activities of daily living became a daily problem. One activity in particular was a fun one for me to help with: I would arrive for our visit at lunchtime and eat lunch with her, hoping that would encourage her to join in. Nope. She quickly learned the most effective response to the spoon moving toward her was to clamp her eyes and mouth tightly shut. I would often try the technique we used with our younger siblings, to recite, 'Here is the airplane, ready to land in the hanger' and sometimes she would open her mouth to accept that one bite. But then the refusal began again. She would occasionally peek out to see if the game would continue, and a little smile would be our reward for pursuing the mealtime in this way. It seemed clear that her sense of humor was intact, even then."

— Bobbi, Daughter

In Late Stage 4, all of the needs of a person with memory loss must be anticipated and it may be challenging to ensure they get enough to drink and eat. They may still be feeding themselves finger foods, but it will require more prompting and eventually needing to be fed and reminded to chew. Words are fewer, and usually there is a great quiet that descends, which often leaves the caregiver wondering, "What are they thinking? What are they feeling? Where are they?" This can be very isolating for both individuals.

The disease affects one's ability to initiate activities and requires caregivers to stimulate and encourage any participation possible without overstimulating the person and causing them to feel stressed. These folks also can fatigue quickly, which in turn affects functioning.

When a person with normal cognition has an illness, they are usually still able to function normally in other areas of the body and act in normal ways emotionally and mentally. They have enough reserves to cope with an illness and still maintain their normal life. When someone has memory loss and is suffering from an illness, it seems to draw on all their resources to try to cope with it or get better. They don't have reserves. We will see sudden dramatic declines in function or changes in behavior with short-term or chronic illness and pain. This in turn leads the caregiver to become a detective, to figure out when the person is actually ill or in pain, because of the lack of communication. The assessment piece is based largely on observation and the person's behavior.

Some folks in this phase become chronically agitated, calling out, constantly moving, resistant to any care. This is the result of all the damage that has gone on over time to the brain and is not at this phase the same kind of emotional expression we witnessed earlier. These are typically misfired messages in the brain and/or self-soothing techniques that require very practical solutions and approaches to help. The immune system is becoming compromised, and frequent infections or recurring illnesses become more common, with increased sleeping noted throughout the day and no impact on rest at night. Sometimes, they will sleep 16–18 hours out of 24. This is the most physical stage.

COMMON BEHAVIORS FOR THIS PHASE

There is a continuation of all the behaviors listed above to a greater or lesser degree, with additional challenges. Repeated movements will be noted, sometimes pill rolling, lip smacking, rubbing something, holding clothes, stripping and layering, rummaging, and some folks need to hold on to something at all times. Bent posture, shuffling gait, falling, and poor judgment all cause greater safety concerns. The person would not be able to recognize or respond to danger. They need cueing, physical assistance with eating, and may not want to chew or swallow items with textures and spits them out. They are incontinent in inappropriate places and will at times interact with bodily excrement without realizing what it is or what should be done with it. They may exhibit combative, aggressive behavior or be very peaceful and calm, easily startled, or difficult to rouse. They may make beautiful eye contact at times or suddenly be able to express a word or sentence. The person may have lucid moments still, but it's very difficult to convey the content due to communication challenges. A person in this stage may like to be physically near, holding hands, sit leaning against the caregiver, or become anxious when they cannot do this, or may appreciate having time physically on their own.

Late Stage 4 Communication Changes
- Silence and stillness pervades—very few words at this point.
- "Of this world, but also of another world".
- Use of nonverbal communication dominates (behavioral communication).
- Responds to environment, weather changes, full moon.
- Repetitive sounds, vocalizations, echolalia more pronounced with some folks.
- Direct one-to-one contact most effective, and may not be able to exhibit a response.
- Physical needs are eclipsing psychosocial needs.
- Increased sleeping and difficult to rouse.

For the Person With the Diagnosis
- Time has a totally different meaning, as they are moving into an internal world, into which it is hard for others to follow.
- The brain has become an ever-thickening filter that is hard to shine through.
- Communication is made with the eyes, body language, simple sounds, and short phrases.
- The desire to sleep is strong.
- The inability to control bodily functions causes different responses, from frustration to completely ignoring difficulties.
- Stillness and quiet descend.
- Letting go, letting go.
- Control has been completely passed into caretaker's hands.
- Having lived a life, they are now returning to the state they entered in—quiet, observing.

For the Caregivers

- Focus on quality of time spent together, rather than quantity.
- Companionship has many expressions. This is a person you can come and just be with, no expectations, no demands. Learn how to be quiet in yourself.
- Focus on review. Speak aloud to the person about the experiences they had, that you had with them, how you felt, how others felt about them. Talk about letting go. Encourage them to talk about how things are being managed and not to worry.
- Look at your own issues around being cared for.
- Giving so much physical assistance can completely exhaust caregivers, in a different way, but just as taxing, as the psychosocial stresses earlier in the disease. Do not judge yourself harshly for needing help; of all the many illnesses, this is the "team approach" disease.
- Consider the idea of "sharing" your loved one with others, rather than feeling you are failing for needing help—others will also learn from the contact with him or her.
- Caregiving assistance may be needed more than ever: utilize available services, such as home care and skilled nursing home placement.

"Although Mom no longer spoke towards the end of her journey, she was always present in the moment. When I would arrive for a visit, even if she had been sleeping, she would awaken with a cheerful, pleasant expression, ready to 'visit' the only way she was able at that point, by being alert and smiling."

— Bobbi, Daughter

Activities that Assist with this Phase

- Play back tapes made of the stories they told (if you have them) or tell stories to them.
- Discuss issues. Forgive them. Talk about your current life.
- Utilize touch—soothing, warm, anchoring, friendly touch.
- Become uninhibited. Sing, take them outside in the gentle sun, wind, and rain.
- Utilize aromatherapy, squeeze fresh orange juice, grind coffee beans, and make coffee or steep tea at their bedside. Eat berries and popsicles, smell roses together, do facials, apply lotion.
- Sit on porches and look out windows.
- Bring animals and children to visit them.
- Make activities of daily living calm, meditative, and serene times together.

Remember: In this stage of the disease, there are losses of what was attained during infancy and early childhood. The focus now shifts from psychosocial needs to physical and medical needs. The person requires more directed stimulus to make contact.

Tips for Resilience

- Maintain a connection to the whole person: the spirit, the part of us that is our essence, and our ability to "be." If we do not experience them as being fully with us, where are they?
- Expanded versus vegetative.
- Focus on meditative, loving service.
- Give the person permission for closure.
- Honor the vessel—it has housed them well and helped them walk through their life.
- Our love is an immortal connection.

FALL PREVENTION

Falls are very challenging. There are fall prevention programs in all elder care settings. Make sure hallways are cleared, with no throw rugs to trip on, that walking paths and stair treads are clearly marked, and that there are hand rails of some type in hallways as well as places to sit and rest along the way. Caregivers need to be trained in how to recognize changes in balance and how to monitor and respond to it. When possible, they should encourage participation in exercise programs. We want elders to maintain muscle strength as long as possible.

For those who use walkers and are starting to have difficulty getting up or sitting down, it is important to enlist a physical therapist or nurse to help model and teach caregivers how these transfers should be assisted. Helping an elder move from one position to another by still recruiting all the muscles the elder should be engaging will create a smooth transfer but also maintain the elder's strength, and keep the caregiver safer from injuries.

Medications can cause some elders to fall, depending on what they are taking. It is important to review medications with the physician, if a change in status is noted with balance or gait.

Families may want to have an occupational therapist or physical therapist come to the home and evaluate the living situation to assess fall risks and ways to try to prevent them. However, we must also acknowledge the reality that falls are unpredictable, especially in a dementia situation. I have had residents gleefully do a sudden dance in a hallway not holding onto their walker, with staff just too far away to catch them. Or residents voiding in inappropriate places and then slipping on the floor, causing fractured hips or head trauma. There have been residents who are territorial or perceive a threat and push someone down, and that person sustains a fracture.

I have seen high-functioning residents suddenly come crashing to the ground on an outing as a result of a new seizure disorder related to how their particular disease progression is affecting their brain. And what do we do? We make the person wear a helmet—someone who still loves wearing matching jewelry and colored outfits and carries her lipstick and purse. She will most definitely refuse to wear one. Other folks who are in Late Stage will not keep a helmet on because, as described earlier, they perceive that glasses, teeth, hearing aids, and other accoutrements are all extraneous. A person in this stage has no sense of why they need these items, so they are thrown aside.

To prevent rolling out of bed, we can move the bed against the wall and create a lump on the outside edge, perhaps using a swim noodle, which makes it is harder for the person to roll over and fall out of bed. We can get a double bed instead of a single bed. We can put a mat on the floor. If the person really lacks insight about their balance, we can get a bed that lowers all the way down to just the depth of the mattress distance from the floor.

In our memory care unit, we try to walk individuals to a point of fatigue, so that when they finally sit down, they don't feel restless and try to get up quickly again. We keep them in an area where staff can see them. In skilled nursing settings, devices can be used to alert staff about when residents try to get out of bed or a chair. All these methods can reduce but not eliminate falls. We know that once most elders begin falling, it is a signal that life is either coming to an end or care levels are going to change. Some elders become fearful after falls, and do not attempt to keep getting up on their own; however, they will accept assistance. This is easier from a care standpoint but sad from a mobility perspective, because all the little movements we do throughout the day are no longer part of this person's repertoire. Physical decline will now accelerate.

It is in this area that I have experienced the greatest challenges with family caregivers. When someone falls at home, somehow this can be integrated by family caregivers. However, if a fall happens under someone else's watch, this seems to be much harder to accept or to process.

I had the same experience myself. When my mother was dropped a couple of times, causing very severe injuries, and I lived at a distance, it was very hard to deal with emotionally. I felt she was so vulnerable, and how could this occur? One time was pure negligence. Someone went off shift, leaving my mother suspended from the highest point of the Hoyer lift over a commode. The person coming into the next shift found her on the floor with a head injury that took nine months to heal.

Lawyers will tell you about negligent situations that should cause a lawsuit. Health departments will tell you about egregious situations that require fines, and perhaps care settings to be closed down. Some caregivers (family and professional) are negligent in home settings or care facilities. This area of care requires that we maintain awareness, work as a team, and have similar goals and problem-solving approaches. It is scary when someone starts careening into door frames, or overcompensates when getting up, or suddenly falls without warning. These things happen even in the best settings, with the best care. Falls are a sad but important example of this issue.

If you find your fury about this issue coming from an irrational place, check in with yourself. We tend to advocate for our loved ones with every ounce of our being. We rage against the onslaught of the disease and lament the changes. We have to be careful about aiming that intensity at the closest caregivers, who are working every day to try to manage the situation. It is important to consider whether you are raging at an innocent bystander, when it is the disease you are angry about. Everyone is learning, and there may need to be some kind of correction or new path pursued. The useful question is what can we all learn? There is a human element in all this. These are changes caused by the person's disease and their reaction to it.

When a territorial person pushes a fellow resident who has approached their door, they do not understand that this person is confused and just looking for their own room. The person pushing is just caught up in the moment and trying to solve a perceived threat and doesn't realize that the other resident is 90 years old and frail, and if pushed will break something. In open environments, everyone should to be able to use all the spaces and move freely.

But when one person is moving into that territorial phase, and someone else comes along who is checking all the door knobs looking for their own room, how do you circulate as a staff member to prevent this interaction every time the person is in their room or the other is on the hallway? We can try to pull elders toward activities that are supervised and create one-to-one opportunities for engagement. We can hang signs and way-finding decorations for the person looking for their room. But even in the best setting, we might not be able to prevent these two from meeting in just the circumstance we are trying to avoid.

A WORD ABOUT CAREGIVER RESPONSIBILITIES

As an operator of care settings, I find denial and blame and unchecked anger in families the hardest thing to deal with. I am grateful this does not come up very often, but when it does, it is typically much harder to handle than the elders we work with—much harder than any staff issues that come up.

My goal is for both family and staff to always work together as a team. As family members, you have known and loved this person we are now just getting to know. How can we work together to improve their quality of life? How can we hold onto aspects of the person's life they enjoyed, and in modified ways still can? How can we focus on their strengths? What can we teach each other? What will you as the family member observe that will be important for us to know? What will we observe that will be important for you to know? How can we share in open dialogue, even if it is painful, to keep working toward the same goals?

Sometimes, families have unresolved issues, and anger or frustration over past events that have nothing to do with what is going on right now that sometimes surface. As caregivers, we may find ourselves in the middle of situations involving siblings and/or siblings and the spouse, an awful experience. It makes providing care in already difficult circumstances almost untenable, and requires a lot of emotional strength to navigate such volatile situations and get back to safe ground.

The only times in the last 25 years when I have seriously pondered leaving this line of work have been when I have found myself caught up in fraught family dynamics. For example, it has on occasion been implied that because I am being paid to do my job I can't possibly care about the residents on a personal level. Such attitudes make me feel negated, painted out of the situation, as if I or my staff were the enemy. Yes, this is my job, and I am doing the best I can, just like the family and the staff. We all play different roles.

When the buck stops with me, though, I accept responsibility. My approach is to pay attention to the canary in the coal mine, with the view that if you stay aware and address the small issues, they won't grow into big scary problems. For example, if we are having trouble sorting laundry and someone has the wrong shirt, let's keep working on improving things. Nor do we want anyone to receive the wrong medication. Managing the details is crucial to managing the big stuff.

Sometimes it is a "systems or procedural" problem; sometimes, it is a training issue; and sometimes, it is an accountability concern. It's crucial to make sure that staff have support, clear guidance of what they are responsible for, training to help them feel inspired about it, and supervision on how to touch in with the right frequency to troubleshoot the situation. Another challenge is that everyone who lives in our building is continuing to change, and just when we feel we have a good strategy, three days or six weeks later it no longer applies.

Most people want to do a good job. We are not throwing pizza here (when the dough sticks to the ceiling you scrape it off and try throwing again). The realm of caring for people is not for the faint of heart. It takes special people to want to do this work, and typically my experience is that staff members are doing the best they can and will continue to learn and grow, as we all do. Sometimes, caring for someone is a huge lesson and an opportunity for personal growth; at other times, the elder is getting the benefit of all the previous learning the caregiver has done.

"For 27 years, I shared in the experience of caring for family members in long-term care facilities: my grandmother, father, and mother. While my father was receiving care, a nurse told me an analogy about memory loss. She said 'Aging is like the rings of a tree. As one ages, all these rings are added over time and get bigger and bigger. But with memory loss, as the person regresses, the outer rings fade and disappear and the focus moves back toward the center of the tree—often to the best and strongest memories in the person's life.'

My mother very much followed that pattern. She always remembered Chicago, Lake Michigan, and her childhood. She forgot who I was. She would ask me who I was, and I would say 'I'm your son.' When she was still speaking, she would answer, 'Don't you wish?'—patting me on the arm. I always worked from where she was and didn't try to convince her. I could visit and be present with her; make sure she was okay but without pressure.

There is a joke I heard. A man visits his father in the nursing home and four elders are sitting together at a table. The son approaches his father and says, 'Do you know who I am?' To which the father says, 'If you don't know who you are, they will tell you at the front desk!' Don't do that to your loved ones; just meet them where they are!

Here is another one for you. A man visits his wife in a nursing home and asks, 'How are you?' She responds, 'It's not so bad, because I am a different person every day.'

I am very grateful my mom's attitude was to accept life as it was, and that she was not sad or fearful. I witnessed some others who were stressed and full of fear about not knowing who or what or where they were and what they should be doing. I was very fortunate that she flowed with things.

A part of our family's values are that you make sure your loved ones are well taken care of. I witnessed it with my grandmother's care, and saw it transition to me through my father's care. Then it was my job with my mother's care. Don't avoid this duty. Don't dump an elder. You will end up in the same boat! What message are you sending to your kids as you work through all this?

I met a gentleman in one of the nursing homes who had moved himself from North Dakota to Boulder.

I asked him, 'Why did you do that?'

'Two reasons,' he replied. 'I don't want to be angry at my kids for not visiting, and I don't want them to feel burdened and be angry about having to visit. This way I am so far away when we see each other it will be special; no need for any anger.'

This was a little extreme, but genius in a way that this elder figured out a way to make sure he got care, but also really didn't want to make his kids responsible for it and created a different option. I am grateful my parents didn't have to make a choice like that, and that we all stuck together through whatever happened. I have no regrets."

— Victor, Son

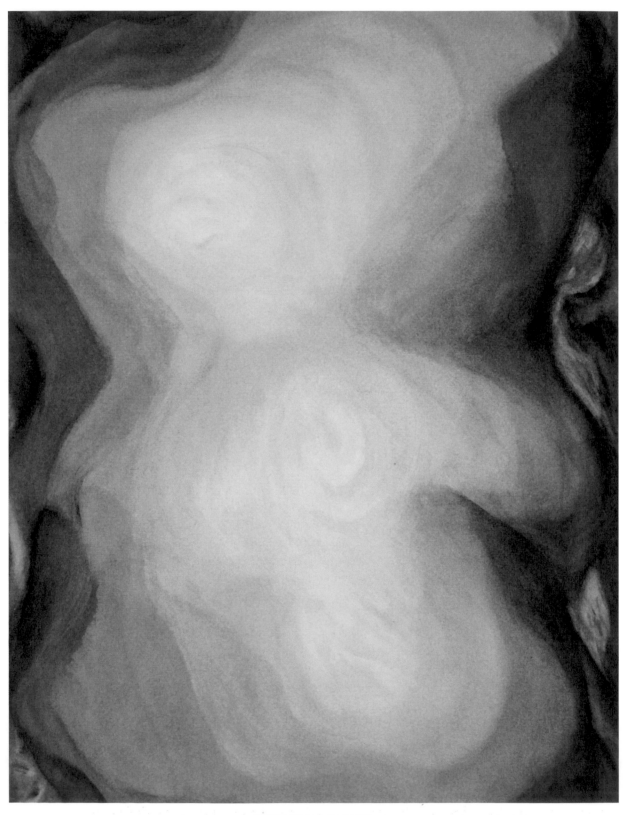

TERMINAL PHASE

TERMINAL PHASE

Preparing for Transitioning – Going Home

How do you know when someone in Stage 4, or Late Stage dementia, is transitioning to a Terminal Phase? This question is difficult to answer. Hospice and Alzheimer's organizations have gotten together and created some guidelines to assist families, caregivers, and medical professionals with sorting this out.

It may be that someone has lost excessive amounts of weight, has had recurring illness such as pneumonia that might be due to aspirating small amounts of food into their lungs, or they have become so immobile they are unable to move normal bodily fluids up and out of their lungs (causing pneumonia). When they are not verbalizing more than 3–5 words a day, are totally dependent for all care, and sleep excessively, these are all signs that the person with memory loss is preparing for their transition. If a person with Alzheimer's takes this journey to its very end, there can be such damage to the brain that a seizure disorder may also occur.

We also see failure-to-thrive cycles. The person dips in their functioning, seems even farther away than usual, and not responding to caregivers in the subtle ways they did before. We see many of the signs outlined above. Everyone begins to prepare themselves, and perhaps hospice is called in. Then in two weeks, or a month, or two months, the person starts to pick up steam again, eating and drinking better, perhaps moving better, participating or interacting more with their caregivers, and graduating from hospice. I have worked with a number of residents who have done this. One comes to mind to whom this happened three different times in five years.

Sometimes, elders genuinely forget to drink, risking dehydration. They may not have been greatly interested in fluids previously, and they keep thinking they have had water, but you know they haven't, as they throw themselves into a severely dehydrated state. In these instances, we have discussed with families trying one round of intravenous therapy (IV) to hydrate them. This may either happen in a hospital because of other issues, or with family, or with staff sitting with them to ensure it gets infused and is promptly removed when completed. We have seen some residents perk up, start drinking fluids again, and not have any more fluid intake problems for a year or two. But if someone moves right back into not drinking, we are probably looking at the person again transitioning into final stages of life. In such cases, we acknowledge our need to prepare ourselves and to assist the person with comfort in their transition.

Most hospice staff agree that dehydration with lack of food intake is one of the most comfortable ways to leave this life. We are so attached to food and the pangs in our stomachs that this may seem hard to believe. We can't imagine being thirsty and not being able to drink. We are active in our life, and that requires sustenance from the earth, fuel to feed our bodies and to energize our endeavors. But what is different in the dying situation is that thirst and hunger are not plaguing the individual. They are disconnecting from these earthly rhythms and needs. The body doesn't want to take in things that add pressure to the systems that are trying to disconnect.

This process is very hard for caregivers, because nourishing is a way we showed our caring. I try to imagine shifts of angels coming in and "spelling" us with their ministrations. We reposition, monitor comfort, and ease physical stress, while they now provide the spiritual nourishment, comfort, and guidance about what's next. We move into being the witnesses, as the angels had been silently doing when we were actively administering our care. Together, we are supporting the transition, this part of life, difficult in its leave-taking but part of the whole story.

Chapter 10

The Boundaries of Quality of Life

In 1987, I was working as a nurse in a nursing home that did not have any specialized program for Alzheimer's. Varying degrees of dementia were exhibited by the residents there—some Early Stage, Middle Stage, and Late Stage.

This is the story of G.

G. lay motionless, her breathing caused her flaccid lips to flap slightly with each exhale. Her body curled in. Rigid flexor muscles had years ago caused her legs to draw up, toes pointed, arms folded tight at her sides. Her hands held washcloths rolled up, to keep her nails from embedding in her palms. She constantly sweated. Her metabolic system was affected by the lack of movement and the liquid food given her through the tube in her stomach. Her medications were crushed and pushed into the same tube with a large syringe. Twice every shift, the nurses would provide routine liquid nutrition and meds, followed by water. She moaned when we turned her.

G. was a Late Stage Alzheimer's patient. She took medications to prevent seizures. We gave her partial bed baths every shift and changed sweat-soaked linens. She had liquid stool, so this also created a lot of linen changes. She had no physical or verbal abilities for communication except her moan . . . and the tears that would gather and seep out of the corner of her eyes and run down her cheeks.

She had been like this for six years. Someone in her family in charge of her care had decided to have the feeding tube put in. No one ever visited her. Someone in the family paid the bill, but no family member had visited for more than eight years. It was excruciating to walk into G.'s room and feel how alone she felt but was not being permitted to let go. Someone somewhere couldn't let her go. For a body to stay tethered to this world by a feeding tube felt really harsh. It felt as if someone else had not owned up to what they needed to do, and G. was giving them a chance day after day to do the right thing. I left employment there and inquired two years later, but the situation had not changed.

I felt I had come in contact with her in order to understand the different qualities of life at all stages and the boundaries of that phrase. G.'s situation can serve as a lesson that despite better care approaches and models of training and environments, there are limits.

There is a natural progression in Alzheimer's and other dementias. We give people a safe space to roam when they start to wander; we redirect this energy and monitor it for safety, instead of ignoring it. When folks stop understanding how to use utensils, we switch to finger foods. We encourage and cajole when elders stop feeding themselves or wanting to eat. We focus on foods they still enjoy, even if that means lots of ice cream. We provide supplements such as nourishing shakes and sit with them and encourage each sip, but we don't force. When someone forgets how to swallow, I personally cannot support fitting them with a feeding tube. The brain is not functioning at this point, and the body is shutting down to allow passage into the transition of death.

It can take the elder the whole 25 years of progression of the disease to finally let go. The underlying will or vitality in their body might be so strong they are unable to disengage on this fundamental level to make the transition out of this life. From our limited perspective, we may not understand what so deeply connects an elder to living that they still actively maintain the thread that holds them tenuously to life. I will speak more about this later, but there can be very strong issues for an elder, related to working out parent/child relationship or spousal roles. Something in these connections may still need time on a soul level to resolve or shift, allowing the elder to realize that it is now time to go on. If that is what it takes, then that is what it takes—everyone must find their own way through this. Validation Therapy, developed through clinical practice with Alzheimer-type nursing home residents, is based on a developmental theory that in old age, when controls loosen, disoriented, very old persons need to express buried emotions in order to die in peace. This final life struggle is called "Resolution."

Validation Therapy

"Validation techniques are based on the principle that when emotions are suppressed they fester and can become toxic. When emotions are expressed to someone who listens with empathy (Validation), the person is relieved. Validation Therapy uses fifteen verbal and nonverbal techniques to communicate with those very old elders diagnosed with an Alzheimer-type dementia and includes a method for forming Validation Groups with time-confused elders. Validation Therapy assumes an attitude of respect for old people diagnosed with a dementia."

— Naomi Feil
    developer of Validation Therapy

It is very helpful if the person with the diagnosis is able to tell you their wishes early on, so that you know how to proceed to honor them. When families must make decisions in the absence of this input, and there are differences of opinion among members of the family, then this can add enormous stress. I try to suggest that families discuss these things in times of wellness, not when crisis or sudden change is occurring. Sometimes urgency is the only motivator of such discussions.

I have also watched family members and professionals trying to cope with a cascade of problems in an elder. In hindsight, after the person's death, all parties could see how with each difficulty, the elder was building up to their transition, just as bouncing on a trampoline allows you to go higher and higher and build the momentum to make the big jump. Problems build and build and become increasingly insurmountable, and you have this desperate feeling, "Could anything else go wrong or get any worse?" And it does, again and again. And then suddenly, after this roller-coaster ride, the person suddenly makes their transition. It seems as though things have to get stirred up enough, be difficult enough, in order to create the momentum that allows the elder to feel "I *am* ready for what's next!" Then off they go.

This is very hard on everyone involved, but there is a strange sense of relief after something like that. You tend to not have any second thoughts about the person, because you don't want them caught in any suffering or pain and are happy they are not dealing with these issues. The storm leads to gratitude for their peace in the aftermath. This can be the case with strong, aberrant behavioral challenges, and also with episodes of illness and falling. I have had this experience a number of times, with everyone doing the best they can. It is heart-wrenching each time.

Early in my career, I worked with a woman who was sprightly. She moved too fast at times and would lose her balance. She had no awareness of losing her balance and would not use walkers or accept assistance. As the disease progressed, the inevitable happened. She fell and broke her hip, had surgery, and while recuperating in the hospital managed to free herself of the restraints, got out of bed, and fell, damaging the repair, necessitating a return to surgery. Afterwards, she came back to the unit and was recuperating in a recliner, with a restraint table across the arm rests, when she managed to free herself again, fell immediately, and broke her other hip. She then went back to the hospital and had that hip repaired, came back to the building, once more got out of her bed restraints—a vest and waist restraint and side rails—and fell, rebreaking the hip.

In the end, the family decided not to send her to the hospital again and initiated hospice. She died within a few days. It was horrible. Did she have a death wish? She was just doing what was normal to her: time to get up and go. I cried and cried each time this occurred again. What was all that about?

Sometime male residents who urinate in inappropriate places slip in their urine and fall, hit their heads, then pass away due to a subdural hematoma, or they break their hip and do not recover. I remember one gentleman to whom this happened. The staff was doing all they could to prevent incidents, taking him to the bathroom at regular intervals and using adaptive clothing to help prevent inappropriate voiding. In between, though, and away from the usual haunts, this person figured out how to get the clothing off, and suddenly we were dealing with a life-and-death situation.

I once had a gentleman move into the memory care unit who was particularly violent. His son, who was probably at his wits' end, failed to mention this during the admission process, and we only discovered it once the gentleman moved in. He had a colostomy bag but did not remember having the surgery to install it. He would wonder what that item was under his clothing and pull it off, flinging it across any room he happened to be in. He did not want to be touched and would assault anyone who moved into his space too quickly.

All of us have a sense of personal space, what is comfortable to us when others enter the space around us. This gentleman's need for personal space was larger than normal, and he felt immediately threatened if others entered or invaded this space. He was a very strong, physically healthy man, so we had to use what I call a "reverse magnet" approach to get near him. We would slowly step into his peripheral space and stay there for a few moments, then he would move slightly away. We would use this to get him moving in a desired direction. It would take about 20 minutes to do this approach. He would get used to our presence and not feel threatened, then we could offer to assist with getting a new colostomy bag in place.

I generally had a good rapport with him, but after a holiday break, I did not spend enough time moderating my approach before trying to contact him and he lunged and tried to strangle me. I would have just tried to flee the room and let him calm down again but another resident was nearby, fortunately unaware of all this, and I did not want the agitated resident to shift his focus to that resident while in his current state. I had to use all of my strength to push back and throw him off balance so that he would land on a bed. I then got in a position where I could pin down his legs with my knees and try to hold onto his arms to prevent him from hitting or grabbing me, while calling out to other staff for assistance.

This took a while, and we were tussling back and forth when I noticed two eyes peering in through the small crack of the door. Then the door slowly closed. To my horror, this staff person was too afraid of the gentleman to get involved and abandoned me. This person also did not immediately go and get help; she totally ignored the whole episode as if it were not happening.

I kept calling out, and finally someone else arrived. My neck was bruised, as well as some ribs, and it took me a while to recover and be able to approach this man again. I had to get over my fear, because folks with dementia are reading your signals, and if you are defensive or setting off fear alarms, they feel this and start getting tense and suspicious. You have to really feel inwardly able to approach in an open and warm way in order to not set yourself up again for the same negative response.

All of the staff was at their limit with this man. This was certainly demonstrated with the clearly passive-aggressive message coming from the individual who had witnessed what was happening but did not offer or seek help. The message to me was, "You assessed him and accepted him to be here, now you deal with it."

We were not able to continue working with this resident. The medications the physician suggested did not work, and it was risking the safety of other residents and staff to continue to have him there. He was transferred to a local hospital and placed in a psychiatric ward, where they tried to help calm his behavior. He was throwing himself against a door in a quiet room and fell and broke his hip. He died within a couple days while they were deciding if they should do surgery or not.

I worked with a woman whose entire stay with us was volatile. She was angry, angry, angry. It never changed, it never softened. It was an incredible struggle. Although word-finding was a challenge for her, as was every task related to daily living, she commented frequently that she should die, that she should not be here. She had a sudden change in status and was moved to an inpatient hospice unit, and during that period she was finally calm. She wanted to let go, but it took two years of fury to get there.

Fortunately, such intense stories are infrequent, but there are still situations that occur with this disease that have everyone running as fast as they can to keep up. They try to do everything they should do, using the best support in the field, yet the care situation can still feel like a tempest.

When souls arrive in this world, what are their stories, what are the beginnings of their unique tale? There is labor to get here. What was your birth story? Was it dramatic, magical, challenging? Or did you arrive with a certain kind of normalcy in the delivery process, the expected series of events seen in so many births? How much of the deep harvesting that goes on throughout this illness also involves the last moments of life here as a review of a person's beginnings. Or is the act of labor once again manifesting itself in the transition? To end this life, there is contraction and pain and a sense of spasmatic force that perhaps enables the individual to leap out of the too limiting space the disease has created for them.

I had a colleague who was riding the bus with two other nursing students when she was a student nurse in a rural area when a woman went into labor right there on the bus! She and her two friends delivered the baby, and the woman named her baby with their three names combined. So when it comes to people with violent tendencies, you ask yourself, "Was there a desperate situation and a surgeon had to reach in and grab the child out? Was there fear for the mother during the birth? Did the mother lose her life at that moment?" There are so many stories that have the expected path and go well, but there are stories that are troubled. Often, we will never know what happened for this individual when they entered this life, but I see some of these dynamics play out with memory loss transitions as well.

....

Chapter 11

Alzheimer's as a Way of Living More Than One Life Experience Within a Lifetime

Let me introduce you to a few exceptional individuals. C. completed her doctorate in Divinity at age 66. L. ran his own business successfully for many years and had degrees in Mathematics, Music, and Law. R. was a brilliant physicist and hung out most of his career with Nobel Laureates. J. was a marathon runner and emeritus professor at two leading universities. D. helped create DOS for computers. W. was a top cancer surgeon.

I have had the good fortune in my nursing career to work with geniuses, linguists, deans, doctors, philosophers, creative thinkers, and artists. They were individuals who had reached incredible personal heights in their careers and their lives, and were either schooled in the traditional way or in the school of hard knocks. All have Alzheimer's or other dementias in common, so clearly this does not support the findings that we can avoid dementia by exercising our brains. These folks were using every extra neural pathway possible. What does this mean? It raises some interesting questions.

Most people recognize President Ronald Reagan's name and know his story. This man had a long and successful career in the public eye, from acting to politics, and made a contribution to the field of Alzheimer's disease by letting the nation know he was afflicted with it. Prior to this, several other celebrities had acknowledged that they suffered from it, but it was Ronald Reagan who made the biggest impact.

Early in 1990, in my capacity as a volunteer for the Alzheimer's Association, I was asked to host a booth at a local health fair, an annual event attended by hundreds of people. Other organizations were set up nearby—the American Heart Association, the American Cancer Association, an audiologist, and so on—and I brought balloons and flowers and had a festive-looking table with fliers and handouts.

Let me tell you what happened. I stood there for seven hours cheerfully greeting people as they passed, but everyone was giving my table a wide berth, as if walking close to it would somehow put them at risk for "catching" Alzheimer's. Only four people actually approached my table all day. The first said, "Oh, my God! What a horrible disease!" and quickly moved on to the next table. The next said, "I know I have it. I can't remember names," and when I asked if she had ever been able to remember names, she said "NO, but I know I have it!" and quickly rushed on. The other two people actually had a loved one with the disease whom they were caring for and were already in contact with the Alzheimer's Association.

At the end of the day, I was feeling somewhat dejected as I was putting my items away, when a woman approached me from the American Cancer Association table. She said, "Don't worry. They all used to treat us and our booth that way. People were very afraid of even saying the word 'cancer.' They thought it was a death sentence, and when someone got diagnosed they often wouldn't tell anyone except the closest person to them—not their children, not coworkers. Now people are not as afraid and realize there can be success stories. Maybe, someday, that will happen with Alzheimer's, too."

When Ronald Reagan was diagnosed with Alzheimer's, people knew the breadth of the life he had led and, with occasional updates from his wife, followed his illness. Nancy Reagan also published a book about their love story and some of the daily notes he had written her throughout their marriage. But what happens sometimes when an individual gets the diagnosis is that there is a feeling of shame and dismissal. "Oh, that is such a shame. They had such a great life." It almost sounds as if the life were wasted because it ended like this.

When it comes to dying, some people fantasize about going to bed and putting their slippers neatly together, pulling the covers up, and just not waking up the next morning. Other folks fantasize about doing something they love, then falling over dead. It might be startling to the rest of the people involved in whatever activity it is, but often mourners come to the conclusion that this is also a great way to go. Other individuals live one kind of extreme life and then, through some kind of accident or injury, experience the opposite extreme: for example, Olympic athletes at the peak of their physical abilities or NFL football players who suddenly become paralyzed or years later suffer dementia.

One such hero was actor Christopher Reeve, best known for playing the role of Superman. Reeve was always an athletic person and enjoyed competitive sports. He suffered a spinal cord injury as the result of a fall while horse riding and never walked again. However, he inspired millions of people after the injury. He put all his energy and celebrity into working toward cures for paralysis. Through his foundation, he pushed for research and raised funds and tried experimental treatments, using himself as a guinea pig, even trying out a new medication that caused him to go into anaphylactic shock. He kept trying new things.

THE ALZHEIMER'S ASSOCIATION

The Alzheimer's Association was established in 1980 in the Chicago area by a group of family members who had loved ones diagnosed with Alzheimer's and found there were no resources regarding the specifics of how to care for someone with this particular challenge. This not-for-profit organization has since grown into a world wide force advocating for individuals with memory loss (Alzheimer's and other dementias), providing education and support for caregivers, friends, and family members, as well as professionals, and supporting research efforts and funding.

He continued acting and directing, raising his young son with his second wife, Dana. He knew he was fortunate to have funds to pay for the best care possible, but he also was a humble and approachable person who wanted to share any inroads into the disease with others and assist patients with fewer means to find ways to access these treatments. He had bad days, too, but his warmth, fortitude, and inner strength are what is remembered.

We are inspired when we see an individual continue to be himself despite devastating setbacks and somehow incorporate the obstacles and still go on. In Christopher Reeve's case, we could embrace the man now confined to a wheelchair because we could still experience him as the same personality through his speech and ideas. Our empathy is engaged as we project onto him our own questions about his situation. How would I handle that? What if I were paralyzed? The sense of personal loss in such a situation can be devastating, and some individuals never make it out of their shock or get over the losses, which linger as anger and bitterness. We all want to be whole. We don't want "bad" things happening to our loved ones or ourselves. But things happen.

When someone takes the experience by the horns and fully engage it instead of avoiding it, something fundamentally shifts in our perception of the situation and also typically how the person will speak about it. They are not a victim anymore. They are able to say honestly, "Yes, I wished this never happened, but I am now aware of. . ." Or, "I understand this. . ." Or, "I believe this. . . and would not have had these insights had I not had these experiences."

I believe it is easier for us to see the blessings in certain situations with positive outcomes, as in cases when an individual comes into this life and it is quickly apparent they have certain gifts and talents, attributes which the circumstances they are born into also nurture. An example of this would be footballer John Elway. He was born into a family that loved football, and his father was a football coach. By the time, Elway was two he was throwing balls with uncanny accuracy, and his mother remarked that even as a child, he could hit anything they identified as a target. This skill kept growing, and as his life unfolded, he became one of the most renowned NFL quarterbacks of our time. Some people are child prodigies whose stories have come down to us through history, such as Mozart. We wonder, how was it possible that this young boy had complete sonatas rolling off his fingers at the age of 13?

In these examples, it is easy to find ourselves saying, "He was destined to do this." In conventional thinking, when someone's life has reached a pinnacle and then something happens to make it go completely in an opposite direction, we tend to judge their life as a failure. What I see, though, is the totality of a life experience—everything that happens is part of our life history, not just selected pieces. It may represent a deeper desire at the level of the soul that with our limited perspective, we cannot understand. Because the Alzheimer's journey renders the person unable to communicate their internal experience, it is viewed as wasted time—indeed, to all outward appearances, Alzheimer's seems to consist of accumulating losses and the inability to function in line with "normal" realities.

But what if this is a rich, deeply meaningful period in the person's life and their understanding of their innermost aspect of themselves? What if it is part of a larger plan, their destiny? What if they are not a victim? What if their essence has been working in this life on the use of mind, the use of the brain, and now they are experiencing vistas and possibilities of this organ that defy description and cannot be conveyed to others? What if the last years of their life are registering on their souls, and that memory has nothing to do with whether they are whole and intact, but experiencing every moment of it, released from their own conventions?

No one in their day-to-day consciousness wants Alzheimer's. That is not what I am suggesting. No one did anything bad to get it, and people diagnosed with the disease are doing the best they can and also wish this were not happening to them. No matter whether you have lived a full and amazing life or a long and modest life, you may still get Alzheimer's. So what is happening?

I believe the soul is whole and intact and busy gathering experiences, learning from this additional toil at the end of life. This is not wasted experience. The soul is busy, busy, busy. This is especially true in situations where there has been excellence in the area of mind or use of the brain. It feels to me that the person is discovering something else by having the experience of opposites. To be very cognitively astute, to use the brain and find self-definition through the use of mind is very normal. There is also an element of seduction in it. If we are truly authentic, we recognize that our physical package changes over time. We recognize that if we define ourselves according to how we looked at 20 years of age we would spend the rest of our life disappointed.

I had an acquaintance once who had been a model. At 32, she thought her life was over—she was actually suicidal. Of course, she was completely stunning, a knockout, the envy of every woman who saw her on the street. But for her, as she looked at images of herself in her early twenties, she might as well have been a hag with no teeth, warts on her nose, and 100 pounds overweight. It was the strangest thing to deal with.

What became apparent in my contact with her was that all her life the only way she had received attention or felt she was getting attention was through her looks. It was not about who she was as a person, or how she felt about things, or what she thought; it was only about her appearance. She felt like an image reflected on the surface of water. Any slight change vibrated and disturbed the image, and she had no idea about her own depth.

The reason she could contemplate suicide so readily was that she felt no connection to her true self. What is that true self gathering as experiences? And what are the challenges we face in our everyday lives that make us stronger and more compassionate, that

"I find myself reflecting about Mom's and my experience from a broader perspective because of the time that has passed. The main thing that strikes me is that Mom was living very much more in the present than she ever had. Before dementia, she was usually thinking about the past or worrying about what the near or far future might bring. She flitted about like a hummingbird, moving from one thing to the next, with her mind clearly not in the present. As she moved deeper into dementia, she seemed to slow down and be much more in the present moment. The future no longer seemed to concern her. Sometimes, something from the past, real or imagined, would surface, and she would get agitated or frightened. Otherwise, she mostly stayed focused on the here and now.

I appreciate the chance to become aware of this change in her. While she was alive, my focus was mostly on the practicalities of what she needed in order to be comfortable, calm, and feel safe, as well as dealing with trips to the doctor or hospital, making sure she had clothes and underwear, etc.—basically the logistics of her life. I can now see a bit of an upside to her condition, whereas before it seemed strictly painful and tragic."

— Linda, Daughter

build our character? Are there individuals you know who strive and challenge themselves constantly in these areas? Or do you run into more individuals who find themselves in situations that create that outcome for them? They were not seeking it, but here it is?

How do we evaluate a life? How do we assess a lifetime and say it was worthy, it was good? As I said earlier, what I hear sometimes in the tone of the statement "Isn't it a shame he or she got Alzheimer's" is that the disease has made the person's whole life null and void. Are we so materialistic that the mind and the brain are thought of as one thing representing the whole person?

We don't feel that way about the heart. We have all these feelings, these emotions, and we say things about our hearts. But typically we don't feel these emotions are literally in the cellular tissue of our heart. When someone has survived a heart attack, we don't say, "Oh, what a shame. He was such a loving and kind person," as if the heart attack stops that kind of emotional expression. Yet our chest swells with feelings, our hearts pound with anxiety or the rush of joy. How can someone have a heart transplant and not be squeamish that all their feelings are going to leave them and the feelings of another are going to invade their system? We know that is foolish. Yet we do not feel that way about our brains, our memories, and the use of our minds.

In his *Principles of Philosophy*, written in the 17th century, the philosopher René Descartes famously stated, "I think, therefore I am," a profound contribution to philosophy and understanding consciousness. In *Being and Nothingness*, written in 1943, Jean-Paul Sartre stated, "If I am thinking, therefore I am, there must be another part of me that is aware of thinking in order to describe 'I am' therefore I am not the 'I am. . .' but something other." What is the "other" in Alzheimer's disease doing?

When I worked with special needs and developmentally disabled children, the families had a lot of concern regarding what kind of life this individual could have. They wanted to understand what was realistic to hope for, while trying to find and do every kind of therapy, service, or program they could to help their child make as much progress as possible. In the back of everyone's mind was, "What will happen when I am gone? How independent will my child be? How vulnerable will they be? Will other people be cruel or take advantage of them in some way?"

In terms of Abraham Maslow's Hierarchy of Needs, what families are addressing is those first crucial bottom layers of the pyramid. They always hope that their special child will feel fulfilled in some way—loved and able to express love, no matter what the level of disability is. There really is a fundamental question about whether this person will get to live a normal life. Will they reach certain hallmarks we consider traditional for a "productive" life?

As I discussed earlier, when I was 20 years old, I lived in the UK and Europe for a year, moving every three months from one Camphill community for special needs individuals to another, all of them modeled on Rudolf Steiner's philosophy of anthroposophy.

"I never cease to enjoy listening to the chitchat that often occurs, especially among the ladies. Whenever there is a tea party, there is a wonderful buzz of conversation. Sometimes the conversation may not make sense to an onlooker, but it's very obvious that they are making loving and meaningful connections with one another. This is especially noticeable at mealtime when a tableful of residents will sit together chatting with coffee long after the meal is over. Life is good for these residents, and they enjoy participating in all that life has to offer during the day. They live very much in the moment, and each moment is a meaningful one."

— Judy Dickinson
  Concierge and Master Gardener
  Program Coordinator

I started out in Norway, helping in a farm community with handicapped adults located by the ocean, 250 miles south of the Arctic Circle. Then I went to England, to a small town near Bristol, and worked in a school for special needs children. Next was northern Scotland, where I lived in four communities located outside Aberdeen. This was the original location of this organization, and there was a special needs children's school and therapy program and, for adults, sheltered workshops and farming.

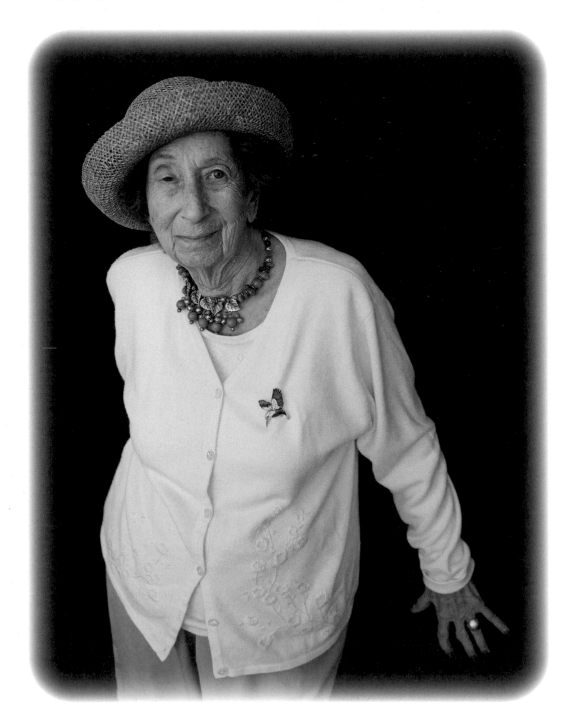

During that year, I knew more individuals with disabilities than I did people without them. This set up an interesting dynamic in my head. I had created this trip in my mind—all the cool things I was going to do, all the amazing people I was going to meet—and I was doing that. But it turned out to be just incredibly hard work, not an ounce of glamour, and the "amazing people" I was meeting ended up being not some Bohemians in a coffee shop but these unique, authentically themselves people with disabilities. They came right at me, straight and real, and welcomed me. They addressed the "me" inside, not the "American girl," the "20-year-old," but the "what-are-you-made-of?" me. I also became aware there was a worldwide network of special people. Just as there is a worldwide network of people who love music, a worldwide network of people who play soccer, and so on.

Each of these endeavors requires certain structures and tools. In special needs settings, it was the rhythms of community, meals being prepared, assistance with whatever part of the day was particularly challenging, the slowly unfolding skills encouraged by coworkers, teachers, and aides.

If you were a musician, it might be tuning your instrument and practicing daily, finding other musicians to play with, being inspired by a particular piece of music. If you loved playing soccer, well, early-morning practice happens all over the world for soccer teams. Each player arrives in cool morning air to hone their skills and tune their bodies, and depending on where the game is being played on the map, calls to each other in that language, dreams about making a perfect score.

Some Thoughts About My Mom, Marie

"I was very grateful that Marie's dementia did not take a mean turn. As she lost more and more of herself, she was only left with the words "I Love You" as her main communication. She would smile and blow kisses. She became very gentle at the end of her life.

Marie was an executive assistant in her professional life. She loved to dress well, wear fabulous shoes, hats, and jewelry. While at memory care assisted living, she employed a personal groomer to color and fix her hair and do her nails. It had always been important to her that she look good. She maintained this habit until very late in the progression of her dementia.

It truly saddened me that she stopped calling me by my name fairly early on. She knew she knew me, and she was always happy to see me, but she did not call me "Laurel." I would have given anything to hear her call me Laurel Belle once again.

On the negative side, she was sent to the emergency room on at least two occasions when she fell down. Those experiences were very frightening and disorienting to her. On the third occasion, I put my foot down and demanded that the nurses not send her out to the hospital and just take care of her there (which they did). It was a much more satisfactory experience for Marie.

Marie was extremely fortunate that she had long-term care insurance and was able to pay for 10 years of assisted living and skilled nursing at the finest facilities in our area. I am eternally grateful for the care she was able to provide for herself."

— Laurel, Daughter

Once, I was stuck in a train station in Milan, Italy, and at 3 a.m., the security guards, the janitorial staff, and the delivery truck drivers to the train station all stopped what they were doing and played an hour of soccer in the middle of the train yards. Whooping and hollering, exhorting stranded travelers to join in and play. At 4 a.m., they patted each other on the back, and all went back to work. It was an unforgettable sight.

What I started recognizing was the validity of these experiences for the individual, and that there were many people engaged in similar efforts all over the planet. Instead of only being aware of one person, or a couple of such people, and having the luxury to say, "Oh, isn't that a shame?" or "Isn't that wonderful?" I knew many people whose reality was different from mine. Their strengths and talents might be different, but they were no less valid or more important to the flow of things all over the world.

Due to the pace and opportunity for service that the Camphill settings provided, I happened to be involved in something that felt very balancing in the rushed and at times egocentric world of our consensual reality. But I could just as easily have been intensely in love with music and having all kinds of experiences related to that. Similarly, there are people all over the world with dementia and memory loss—it is just another experience amid myriad experiences that human beings can have during an individual lifetime.

Think back to periods in your own life that now feel almost like another lifetime— childhood felt different from teen years, young adulthood different from middle age, and so on. Some individuals make enormous changes in their lifestyles and feel that that earlier person was not who they really are, and now they are more themselves. A butterfly's metamorphosis offers something else to think about, as a caterpillar can't recognize itself as a butterfly. Others may feel that they are evolving, growing, and shedding outer layers, yet still mostly look like themselves. There are elders I know who reflect these approaches in their aging process.

If we need to look for an additional blessing, many individuals with Alzheimer's attained all the outward hallmarks of success that society expects of us. They grew up, completed schooling, held jobs, had careers, met others they could share dreams and a life with, raised families, had hobbies and interests, volunteered, mentored others, and shared their wisdom and humanity. By way of contrast, the potential in life that most of us think of as "a normal life" is something many of the special needs children at Camphill would never achieve.

This brings me back to Ronald Reagan. What was so touching to me after his death was the full state funeral that was held, befitting his status as a former US President, yet in the minds of many members of the public at odds with who he had been in the final decade of his life due to Alzheimer's disease. Folks who might not have normally thought about it found themselves thinking about what it must have been like for this man who had been involved in so many life experiences yet could no longer consciously recall them. Because people were so familiar with stories about Reagan, this could not be so easily dismissed. It was a breakthrough to have news media ask about the status of Reagan's dementia in the last years and months, and for the public to engage in a dialogue about this difficult process. It really helped to bring this disease out into the open and not be treated like the leprosy of our time. To have the entire country stop for a moment to observe the passing of a life—a life full of many experiences, including Alzheimer's—and to have that person honored for the entirety of their life was a final tribute to all people living with Alzheimer's disease.

[The following letter is reproduced exactly as written and was obtained through the archives at the Ronald W. Reagan Presidential Library & Museum. http://www.reaganlibrary.net/]

Nov. 5, 1994

My Fellow Americans,

I have recently been told that I am one of the Americans who will be afflicted with Alzheimer's Disease.

Upon learning this news, Nancy & I had to decide whether as private citizens we would keep this a private matter or whether we would make this news known in a public way.

In the past Nancy suffered from breast cancer and I had my cancer surgeries. We found through our open disclosures we were able to raise public awareness. We were happy that as a result many more people underwent testing. They were treated in early stages and able to return to normal, healthy lives.

So now, we feel it is important to share it with you. In opening our hearts, we hope this might promote greater awareness of this condition. Perhaps it will encourage a clearer understanding of the individuals and families who are affected by it.

At the moment I feel just fine. I intend to live the remainder of the years God gives me on this earth doing the things I have always done. I will continue to share life's journey with my beloved Nancy and my family. I plan to enjoy the great outdoors and stay in touch with my friends and supporters.

Unfortunately, as Alzheimer's Disease progresses, the family often bears a heavy burden. I only wish there was some way I could spare Nancy from this painful experience. When the time comes I am confident that with your help she will face it with faith and courage.

In closing let me thank you, the American people for giving me the great honor of allowing me to serve as your President. When the Lord calls me home, (sic) whenever that may be I will face it with the greatest love for this country of ours and eternal optimism for its future.

I now begin the journey that will lead me into the sunset of my life. I know that for America there will always be a bright dawn ahead.

Thank you, my friends. May God always bless you.

Sincerely,

Ronald Reagan

Ronald Reagan

....

Chapter 12

Alzheimer's as a Way of Allowing Matriarch and Patriarch Roles to Transition to the Next Generation

In some families affected by a loved one's memory loss, I have noticed a dynamic occurring that offers family members time to prepare themselves for the next phase, and ultimately for the departure of their loved one. This is especially marked in situations where the matriarch or patriarch has been particularly influential in the family.

I first noticed this when I worked in Philadelphia. Large families would visit the elder in the facility, and it was clear that the adult children were still seeking direction from the elder. Initially, this was a sound approach, as that person still had many opportunities to express their lucidity in Early Stage dementia. As the elder progressed in the disease, though, this was less and less productive, and the floundering children were forced to make their own judgments and decisions.

This was terrifying to some of these adult children. They did not trust themselves and felt the world was only manageable with input from their parent. If the elder had an autocratic style, this was even more paralyzing for the child. The transition includes finding the emotional connections that are still palpable, appreciating them, and recognizing when an elder is providing a pearl of wisdom, an insight that comes zinging out of the confusion, even as the adult children increasingly are forced to look to their own authority in decision making.

A healthy person does not want, of course, to give up their independence, and elders want to stay in control of their affairs. Some elders choose to delegate things that no longer hold their interest or that feel like a burden, and in some families, this is easily taken up by other members. Some sibling groups I encounter divide up their roles in the family at this point—one may be maintaining the property, another addressing the bill paying and accounting, another being a liaison to the physicians and handling the medications, while another may make regular visits and provide meals or housekeeping. Some elders, however, refuse all such support and view it as interference, and trying to "overrule" a parent can be a scary thing. If the parent was perceived as infinitely wise and always right, the need to take charge can be particularly confusing and stressful.

Because dementia is insidious, it changes things slowly over a number of years. The person with dementia is often trying to conceal their challenges, and while the children may have been aware of lapses for a long period of time, they may not feel compelled to act until the shift becomes too dramatic to ignore or deny. This faltering in the elder forces adult children to step into their own power. They hesitate, can't figure something out, don't understand what they should do, but eventually every realm in which the elder was in sole charge is taken over by members of the next generation.

Over time, this transition becomes more normal, understandable, and incorporated into the adult child's capabilities. Some family members have felt this to be an important opportunity. If the person had suddenly died, from a stroke or heart attack, for example, the devastation and disarray in the family would have felt insurmountable and, as one person said to me, "unrecoverable." With this situation, the steps involved in what is needed next are clear. Although the caregiver may feel the situation is entirely about the elder's needs, it is actually the elder helping the caregiver with their personal growth and sense of autonomy.

Some children have their own problems with aging and have rigidities that make it challenging to adjust to their parent's new situation, and not all parent-child relations are resolved when the parents reach their senior years. For example, I once worked with two adult daughters, aged 80 and 83, respectively, and their mother with dementia, who was 99 years old.

In this particular instance, the daughters moved their mother to our facility but did not bring a single personal item from her home. Upon arrival, the mother, who had lived in her apartment building for 40 years, was clutching just her purse and door keys. (She was the person I gave as an example earlier of trying to find her old apartment but nothing looked familiar in her new setting.)

Her daughters were too overwhelmed by their own lives to be able to deal with their mother. To avoid having to sort through her things, they took what they wanted out of the apartment and had a consignment company come and haul the rest away. They had no idea it might be helpful for her to have something she recognized in the new facility. When I tried to discuss this with them, they immediately shut me down saying, "She doesn't know anything; it doesn't matter."

This elder was a sprightly, warm, and lovable person. She immediately befriended anyone who came her way. She loved music and loved to dance. She performed classic theatrical tap dance routines, where the person does tap steps while swinging their arms, coming forward at the end, one arm up, one arm down, one foot forward, one in back. She would actually leave the ground, which made all of us jump the first time she did it, worried she would fall. This deeply embarrassed the daughters, and they would immediately tell her to "Stop it. Sit down. Don't be so stupid." This was hard to observe, because what the elder loved doing was immediately squelched by her daughters.

As the disease progressed, this elder started reacting to the overstimulation of the day and all the people and activities in the unit by reversing circadian rhythms: she slept all day and stayed up all night. The night shift staff spent most of the night with her, as she enjoyed the one-to-one time this provided in the quiet of peaceful hours. She was tiny and had not had any falls, but we did not want to use medications to try to reset her body clock to daytime because she seemed so happy with this routine, and it was not harming her or anyone else. She would wake up for certain meals, snacked during the night, and her weight and overall health were stable.

The daughters visited rarely, but one day they came in and said they were going to move her. On her discharge papers, we explained her routines and how staff was working with them. To check in and see how she was doing two weeks later, I called the new facility where she had been moved to and was told she had died. Apparently, staff had used strong sleeping medications to get her hours "right" again and she immediately started falling. She had nine falls in 11 days and ending up with a subdural hematoma, which ultimately caused her death. No one had stopped the medication usage, even with the awareness of all the falls. It was tremendously upsetting. I also do not have any idea what it was like to be brought up by this mom. I wondered about the attitudes they displayed today—what was a direct legacy from her, and what was of their own creation?

Here is a more specific example of this issue.

G. had been a schoolteacher in elementary schools her whole career and had raised five children. When I started working with her, G. was incredibly nice to other elders on the unit, cooperative with care, and loving toward staff and toward her daughter, who lived nearby and would visit occasionally. Every now and then there would be a sudden mean, even frightening reaction to something going on with her care or on the unit. We worked hard to identify the triggers for these reactions and to consciously avoid them. No one else from her family would visit. The daughter who came was very cool and kept her distance and would tend to physically view her but not want to interact with her. If her mother saw the daughter she would approach her, try to hug her. It was apparent that this made the daughter very uncomfortable.

We had worked with this family for about two years, when I (naïve and always hopeful) asked if there was any way I could help her with her relationship with her mother. She drew back sharply and stated, "You have no idea who my mother really was, or is. You have no idea of the harm she caused us all. To the outside world, she was the wonderful teacher. Everyone thought that she was a wonderful mother . . . but behind the closed doors of our home she was a monster. She physically and emotionally abused all of us for as long as we can remember. It was excessively cruel, and all of us bear deep, deep scars. I am not like her, and I come here to check on her. I provide a good setting for her to live out her life, and I will not be cruel and abusive in return to her. She is my mother. She bore me into this life, but I am the only one of my siblings that can manage this, and I barely manage. I know you are trying your best, but you have no idea, and this is not going to heal or get better. This is the best I can do."

This situation was very educational to me, and I appreciated her candor and guidance. It is true that I had no idea what life had been like for her, and it was information that changed how I viewed the situation and stopped my judgments. I was feeling the daughter was distant and didn't visit enough and wondered why she wouldn't hug her mom.

This brought me abruptly to clarity. I am involved in people's lives during their difficult process, and they are sharing in my life. We are learning from each other. I have to really pay attention to when added support or information is helpful, but not judge or get overly invested in what I wish would happen. "Being of service" can mean advocating and jumping into action, but can also be balanced with knowing when to let something flow and when to let go and be receptive to allowing, which are also parts of service.

I will now tell staff this story when I begin to hear some sort of judgment being conveyed, in order to remind everyone that this is not our place and we are working on learning how to support unconditionally. Generally, staff has a sense of what the progression of the disease is going to look like. They participate in a culture within the residence that can become impersonal at times, or colored by people's ineptness in communicating, or lack of consciousness in how they carry and convey themselves. All of this can have a big impact on a family.

In some facilities, an elder can arrive and seem to be absorbed into the building, as if the staff owns them. It is hard to describe. The challenge for us as staff is to recognize that this person has been part of a family group, has influenced the group, still views themselves within the context of that group, and they have all been on a long journey together. As caregivers, we are coming onto the scene very late in the game. We have knowledge of things that might be helpful, and we want that to be used where needed. But it is extremely important to also avoid falling into any sense of superiority.

We are being given some fundamental lessons in respect for personal process and when to mind our own business. We involve families in a team approach, so that they feel absolutely necessary to this new group dynamic yet can do it in a way that allows them to be as involved or as uninvolved as they wish. Sometimes dementia allows specific family members space to process things in their own way, in their own timing. We are witnesses, and this is an honor. There is a profound richness that touches everyone's life when this balance is struck.

Gracious Acts

Walkers
Wheelchairs
Dementia

Do not define
Identify

Humanity

Peony, whose first language
is Chinese,
Took my hand and found
the elusive words,
"Your mother has wisdom."

— B. Valerie Peckle, Daughter

....

Chapter 13

Alzheimer's as an Opportunity to Be Cared For and Share the Role of Time Keeper

Flossie rode the wagons west! In 1987, when I started working with this particular resident, she was 105 years old. She had been born in 1882. Imagine the changes she had seen in her lifetime. At 18, she witnessed the turn of the century, and at 32, the outbreak of World War I. When she was 52, she experienced the Depression, and at 63, World War II. She probably thought that by the time she reached 80 years of age, she would no longer grace this life, yet here she was in 1987, still among us. She was in amazingly good health—somewhat hard of hearing, with slight visual impairment—and looked like a 60-year-old, her skin soft and smooth and on her head beautiful, thick, snowy white curls. She was at times delusional.

We don't need to bury time capsules and dig them up later to interact with the past—we just have to look around and catch it from the timekeepers around us. Literally, if you draw in close, you can feel the sparkling dust of other times swirling around such people. What gems, what richness! My bias is evident: I believe everything that gets old gets better.

Where do our experiences go? Do they convert through a series of rhythmic processes in the brain to memory, a highly condensed storage area? Or are we living products of our time? I always find it fascinating to experience people who are somehow stuck in a certain time frame. It might be something as simple as a hairstyle not changing for 40 years, or furniture in a house being unchanged since 1962. Is it finances? Is it because of a certain focus of consciousness, which felt comfortable in that era and continues to live there?

An example for me was observing the plain Amish in their deliberate effort of nonparticipation in the fancy world of progress. Some of this can translate for people to stability, comfort, and security. As a child visiting my grandparents' houses, I found a reassuring "sameness" from things remaining in their familiar places—that all things had stories attached to them, which I heard over and over, gave me a connection to family beyond my immediate experience and gave me an understanding of lineage and legacy. Those feelings allowed me, as an adolescent growing into adulthood, to experiment or take risks without losing a fundamentally grounded part of me. I was part of the river flowing forward—a river whose source ran many, many generations back.

I frequently visit private homes when I do assessments. Sometimes I can "feel" a certain era in our nation's history has greatly impacted the person or family. Similarly, certain personal experiences can linger in the space. Sometimes, the two intertwine.

I visited a home where one spouse was caring for the other. They had lost all three children to a fatal genetic childhood disease. The sorrow was that the children did not show symptoms until around six years of age, so they had had all three children before they realized all of them had the disorder. Now the mother of the family had Alzheimer's, and the husband was caring for her. It felt incredibly cruel that the remaining spouse would be dealt such a hard fate. But what was more painful was to be in the house and feel time was holding still in the era when the children had been alive. I could feel it in every room. Then I realized the children were indeed still there, not the way the space reflected but through invisible support. They were available out of body, out of illness, to provide loving constant support to the couple and their situation. There was no way this caregiver could have provided care as long as he had without them. I cried all the way home from this assessment.

Flossie had memory loss in the clinical sense. Her short-term memory was very short. Her ability to recall new information lasted about 10 minutes, but certain things in her long-term memory she remembered clearly and could speak of them vividly. She also could be delusional and hallucinate. In other words, from an Alzheimer's perspective, she would be reexperiencing the areas of memory she still retained and would be reliving them, projecting them on the here and now.

Occasionally, this proved to be especially exciting to her and those around her. She would be calmly sitting in her wheelchair and she would physically jump in a startle response and whoop, crying, "Whoa! Hold on! These horses are scared! They bolted. Oh, saints above, we're gonna lose everything in the wagon. Whoa! Hold up! Uncle Bob's comin'. Come on, come on, catch up! Grab ol'Baron! Get'em to slow. That's it, that's it."

All of this was being physically played out by Flossie as she jerked about in her wheelchair, holding on to her invisible reins for dear life until the horses finally slowed. Flossie had come west on a wagon train to Colorado. There was never any particular cue we could figure out that would prompt these active recollections, but we were along for the ride and got glimpses of the life of many years ago brought vividly into the present.

Newscaster Tom Brokaw's book *The Greatest Generation* suggests what is special about the generation that came of age during the Great Depression and the Second World War was that it was not only united by a common purpose but common values: duty, honor, economy, courage, service, a love of family and country, and above all responsibility for oneself. He tells the stories of many men and women, heroes and heroines, whose everyday lives reveal how this generation persevered. Without whining or complaining or feeling entitled they applied themselves to create interesting and useful lives and build the modern America we have today.

In working with these elders, I find that the values that Brokaw mentions remain even when dementia is present. I have worked with many elders who want to report for work every morning. They feel responsible for their families and have a dignity and steadfastness that is unwavering, a belief in hard work, applying oneself to solve problems, a kind of optimism about life, and moving forward through difficulties. Even how someone expresses their gratitude nonverbally, in very late stages of this disease you can feel the deepest parts of the elder still being conveyed.

This is part of the reason why I find the work I do so incredibly rewarding. I get to be in the presence of these great individuals, who are often humble and modest, and in the time we spend together, soak up some of the greatness that defined them. I hope their example is contagious. In fact, at times I find myself feeling displaced, as if I should have lived then instead of in the strange times we live in now. This may be an additional element to the sense of kinship I feel.

I don't typically perceive chronological age as relevant in my day-to-day dealings with residents. At any given time, a person may respond and react from, say, their 26-year-old, 40-year-old, or six-year-old self, but this may change from moment to moment. My job is to stay fluid enough inwardly to know where we are; I do not use the dear etched wrinkles or age spots on the outer package as a guideline. It is one of the gifts of Alzheimer's that chronological age is really irrelevant.

The other gift of interactions in this setting is that I am often aware of the progress that has been made in modern times with respect to our freedoms and biases. Some of what happened in the past was not optimal. Take women being limited in their job choices. I have worked with many female teachers and nurses, and years ago, there was some strange perception that if you married you could not continue working and would need to raise your family.

"It may be historically premature to judge the greatness of a whole generation, but indisputably, there are common traits that cannot be denied. It is a generation that, by and large, made no demands of homage from those who followed and prospered economically, politically, and culturally because of its sacrifices. It is a generation of towering achievement and modest demeanor, a legacy of their formative years when they were participants in and witness to sacrifices of the highest order. They know how many of the best of their generation didn't make it to their early twenties, how many brilliant scientists, teachers, spiritual and business leaders, politicians and artists were lost in the ravages of the greatest war the world has seen."

— Tom Brokaw,
The Greatest Generation

But what if you were a great multitasker? Managing work and home life would have then been a great extension of your abilities. What if you found you couldn't have children? Because you were having sex in a sanctified union you still couldn't go back to work. That must have been very frustrating to some.

I love good manners and the art of being gracious, which I definitely learned from my grandmothers and mom. However, in the case of one of my grandmothers, she had underlying judgments that were traditional and unresponsive to changing times. She had grown up in Washington, DC, during an era when there were clear class distinctions, racial bias, and harsh social rules about what was acceptable and what crossed a line. She was horrified when I began working with disabled children. She said that, in her time, babies born with disabilities were silently placed in a dresser drawer, left to die, then removed. This was particularly biting because we had someone with some special needs in our immediate family. My grandmother was a generous person but had this side to her that was rigid and sometimes mean, too.

I have worked with many elders from my grandmother's generation who, with the loss of impulse control, start screaming racial epithets at the dear staff who help them most. We can talk about being like ducks, that the oil on our feathers can let this raining shower of insults just wash right off. Ordinarily, we know this level of bigotry is left unspoken, but the dementia can intensify fear, which makes elders respond this way, so we wonder how to lessen their fear. Or this may be some old stuff that they are having a chance to expunge, and in some cases have new experiences that someone different from them actually can end up being the person they seek out most to be with.

"Minding the company store" is another concept that was valued in our recent past. Many of our elders experienced working for many years for the same company or same location, perhaps in farming or other trade. The belief that "I am the steady support for my family" was a wonderful stabilizing factor in many homes. But what if someone really wished they could be doing something else? What if they had an absolute longing in the core of their soul but because of these social norms could not or would not risk shifting to something else for fear of destabilizing everything they were maintaining? This must have been deadening to some individuals and not the healthiest option for their passions.

Thankfully, we have more options to create our own path in our life today. The Silent Generation laid the groundwork for the Baby Boomers. As a massive demographic group at each stage of their development they have made impacts that have changed our society. Author and public speaker Ken Dykwald speaks to this reality in his book *The Age Wave: How the Most Important Trend of Our Time Can Change Your Future*. Individuals in the Baby Boomer generation have changed careers, had second families, taken sabbaticals, traveled before retirement, and altered our perceptions of aging. As much as I can look back and wish we still maintained a little formality, I am grateful that my generation has had more choices about what we individually can choose to do. My hope also is that diversity will continue to be less threatening, and we will learn to appreciate differences in cultural background and life experience in others as interesting additions to our own perceptions. I look forward happily to the dying out of bigotry and racism.

Honoring our elders with compassion, appreciating the good and the not so good in this process, we have frequent opportunities to bring to bear the best of ourselves. We have the chance to manifest gratitude and appreciation for those who went before us, who created the foundation of our lives, and to honor them. This disease peels back layers of artifice and gets right to the nitty gritty of any issue. It de-

"We're usually so busy in our lives, so quick to assess and measure ourselves and our actions. After being with my friends with dementia, I come away as if I've gone to another land where those typical tools for navigating around each other are diminished and don't play such a primary role. Instead, there's a larger sense of acceptance of each other just as we are. It's very palpable."

— Ellen
Geriatric Case Manager

mands our constant focus and attention. It brings out strengths in each of us that we didn't know we had and highlights areas where we still have farther to go. In the deepest sense, the elders we care for allow us to have this experience.

> "It is a privilege to work at the salon with this population. I am fully present, and with a loving intention focus on the task at hand. Always doing the best of my ability. The residents deeply appreciate this attention to their beauty needs and always surprise me with expressions of deep gratitude. Once after working on Glenna's hair, she came back to the salon a little while later, beaming. Something she had just read in a Reader's Digest moved her to express to me her deep appreciation for what I do for her in the salon and to express how much she enjoyed our friendship and how meaningful it was to her. Deep emotion poured from her heart. We were both in tears. I was profoundly touched."
>
> — Cathy Poole, Licensed Cosmetologist

....

Chapter 14

Alzheimer's
as a Way to Escape
an Unbearable Situation

Over the years, I have witnessed some situations with dementia in which it feels as if the person could not find a way out of a personal relationship that was very toxic to them, and because of their way of thinking about the situation, these individuals could not shift the dynamics into something different. The problem could be either in the way they handled the circumstances or in their inability to remove themselves completely as a way of honoring their own needs or desires.

I do not know, so must respect the intimacy within a relationship that only the two parties experience. However, although I have not been present in the person's life prior to the dementia diagnosis, I have noticed recurring themes arising, as families describe the types of patterns their loved one exhibited in their primary relationship. They may, for example, describe a kind of personal sacrifice, a subjugation of the person's desires and passions. Some family members make statements like, "I wish my parents would have divorced," or "I wish my mother would have sought professional help for her mental illness, but instead my father dealt with the brunt of it his whole life."

There is a deadening quality to living with something that feels like a distortion that is never openly acknowledged; it's like living with the unacknowledged elephant in the living room year after year. In such situations, responsibility is never redistributed. The self that knows the truth may rise up in small efforts, but by never fundamentally changing the dynamics, it becomes a smaller and smaller voice in the equation.

We know from dementia research that changes can occur in the brain up to 20 years before an outward sign of the disease is exhibited, and we know that depression can be a risk factor for developing Alzheimer's disease. If a person has been struggling for years with an underlying depression this increases their vulnerability to dementia. Sometimes, relationships can create a kind of festering toxicity, which contributes to this vulnerability.

I want to be clear that I have worked with many elders with memory loss who are in strongly committed primary relationships. For such couples, their relationship has been a healthy challenge. Their commitment to each other has helped them get through rough times, so that, looking back, they have a sense of fulfillment, joy, and pride that they remained together. It was socially expected that if you married you stayed committed to that relationship.

With divorce rates rising, our more recent generations long to figure out how their elders did that. We will have different issues to struggle with in our generation, but this idea that you stand by your partner, you hang in there no matter what, can in some situations be very damaging to an individual's psyche. If you lived with an elephant in your living room, couldn't you imagine at some point you would run screaming from the room? When the person is so committed, with their rational side subjugated over many years, the inner conflict results in a need to vacate. Since this cannot occur on a physical level, the spirit no longer feels comfortable penetrating and trying to shine through, so it becomes vulnerable to demented states of mind.

In an era when a commitment meant staying together no matter what, and folks did not readily go to a psychiatrist to get assistance with mental health issues, some individuals have found themselves in untenable situations. Let me tell you, for example, about one couple I worked with who met in Europe in the late 1960s.

No one knows much about the wife's true history because this woman had a compulsive need to be important, which manifested in constant revisions of her life history, accomplishments, and accolades. She most likely had a personality disorder, which in the family was viewed as a tendency toward the eccentric. They were so used to coping with this "normal" that they did not recognize how far off the beaten track of normal they were. The woman's only child fled to a teen marriage to get herself out of the situation.

In an era when a commitment meant staying together no matter what, and folks did not readily go to a psychiatrist to get assistance with mental health issues, some individuals have found themselves in untenable situations.

As the years passed, this entrenchment deepened and became more and more intolerable. The wife could be very loving and kind but also very cruel and excruciatingly critical. These distortions and arbitrary mood swings left other family members constantly off balance. The wife was skilled in playing the victim, and wielded it like a club. When I first came into the situation, both the wife and husband were suffering from memory loss and social services were threatening to put them under state care. At that point, the daughter stepped in. After a stressful period of daily visits, she was finally able to get them moved, under competent geriatric care, to our residence. In this situation, medications to manage the mental health issues were needed and brought a significant amount of calm to the disruptive and trying dynamic.

The husband and wife were both chain smokers. To accommodate their needs, we created a hard-and-fast schedule that allowed them smoke breaks outside at two-hour intervals; we refrained from encouraging them in their smoking but did not stop it from occurring. Initially, the couple was very focused on this routine, but since they were now in a communal living situation, with caregivers and lots of activities going on, they started to be distracted and did not initiate the smoke breaks. Eventually, months went by without them going outside to smoke a cigarette.

The wife's pattern of controlling her husband and their activities continued for some time. She would demand to be wheeled, ask him for help, be loving, then suddenly switch to yelling at him. She would start a discussion and escalate his paranoia, then solicit help to "calm him down." She tried to dominate others living in the same area of the building, constantly challenging others' relationships and causing "triangulation"—in other words, pushing people to take sides by becoming upset at some invisible offense and then in the height of the drama, absolving herself of any connection and reverting to a superior tone or stance. She was particularly deft with her spouse, pushing him away and pulling him in. It was hard to witness.

I worked with staff on looking beyond this posturing to the detectable frailty in the wife's sense of self, suggesting that it had been her only option for coping in our stressful world without professional help. She did not have the ability to recognize how psychologically damaging her actions were to others. I wanted both individuals to be able to experience support and a sense of peace and acceptance.

Working with the wife was a bit like trying to comfort a spine-covered sea urchin, but I still felt this could occur at some level. It is my fundamental belief that people with dementia are managing the best they can. And although this person had a dual diagnosis and often required approaches that were more aimed at behavior than dementia, I still lived in hope.

When I find a care situation with an individual particularly challenging, I use the following four criteria to address it:

1. **A problem is a solution we haven't found yet, so put on the detective hat and ponder.**
   - Is it physical—a pain, a discomfort, or too much vitality that doesn't match the situation?
   - Is it emotional — a longing, a loss?
   - Is it a recent feeling or was it buried, now excavated—a long held and perhaps never expressed emotion? How can we help the person explore this in safe ways?
   - Is it spiritual—a crisis of identity, an unexpressed potential, a sacrifice, or offering of some kind?
   - Is this person a teacher who we should awaken to—in other words, it is not about them; they are shining a light on us and something we need to learn?

2. **We always want to channel energy instead of stopping it.**
   - How can we create opportunities to redirect actions and behaviors in a way that helps them be fully expressed and expended in positive ways?

3. **We want to highlight strengths, not spotlight weaknesses.**
   - How can I help this person finds ways to use their skills, be appreciated for their gifts, and not embarrassed by what has become difficult?

4. **Sometimes slowing down is the fastest way to get something done.**
   Often, what we need to do is literally slow down our actions in order to help the person process what we are doing and find better ways to do what is needed. Another aspect of this is to get quiet and really listen, check in with intuition, observe without expectation, and soften the lens with compassion to see things in new ways.

We began to focus on ways to create spaces for her husband to get a break from all this. If she was napping, we encouraged him to come to activities on his own. The staff worked on getting him out of the building on outings. The wife started to have more challenges with her health and was allowing staff to assist her more with her needs. This also helped her feel supported and cared for.

Then an interesting thing occurred. The husband started getting clearer in his thinking. He began remembering names and staying on track with time without cueing. His humor started to bubble up, and his artful teasing amused and surprised all who came in contact with him. He was doing a better job with shaving and dressing and was not sleeping for endless periods during the day. He started seeking out other female companionship. He would check in on his wife but started declaring that he had moved on, that he should have done this years before, and that they were now divorced but could be friends. The wife became aware of his interest in other residents and informed me one day that they had been divorced for a year and four days, but that he was still her lover whenever she demanded it; she didn't need to know the details.

As I write this, the wife has gotten gentler in her mood swings and critical moments. She now enjoys activities on her own more, and although she will still yell at folks, this is far less frequent or intense. This couple on their own could not find a way to disentangle themselves and allow more healthy mental space between them. They needed a team and a living situation that facilitated this change to create an opportunity for healing. If the husband is able to have a period that truly brings him happiness and levity so that he can feel mentally more engaged, even for a short period of time, then it feels worth the struggle. Ultimately, the dementia will not be cured, but the ways it has progressed for this man appear strongly altered by the change in dynamics.

Years ago, I worked with a woman who had a very unfortunate chain of events occur in her life as she was about to leave the family home. She was an only child and became engaged to a gentleman who was only able to find a job in a distant town. As the couple prepared for their wedding, the woman's father became critically ill and she had to help her mother with his care. The financial situation was not good, so she had to get a job to help her immediate family cope and had to put off her wedding.

For eight years, the woman's fiancé waited. He continued to work in the distant town, trying to establish a comfortable financial future for them both. Then, unbelievably, her mother became ill. A few months later her father passed away, but she continued to try to manage the situation with her mother. She and her fiancé wed, and she and her mother moved in with the spouse in the distant town. The newlywed cared for her mother for five years before the mother passed away. The woman had about two years of family life without illness, and had a child late in life, before her husband became ill and died. Left to raise her son alone she coped the best she could, but she increasingly came to feel that life was unfair and harsh and that she would never experience happiness.

I met this woman late in her life, when memory loss was making it difficult for her to remain living on her own. Her son did not have an easy time relating to her, and her angry isolation seemed impenetrable. Her dementia felt like a last resort, silently communicating the message: "Don't make me responsible for anyone else. Take care of me. Take care of it all. I can't cope. I can't cope!" Over the months and years I worked with her, however, she became far lighter in her humor and way of relating, now that all the mundane things were handled by someone else and she was safe from the threat of life laying yet another devastating burden on her.

The last story in this regard is a man who married his wife just after World War II. She had serious issues with depression, which had plagued her throughout her life, and was very demanding. Their relationship spanned years and years of co-dependent dynamics. The husband was successful in his career, which provided a stable home for their children to grow up in and which allowed them to go on successfully with their lives and career. But he had difficulty with patience and angered easily, and this was a source of tension in the family: the mother's demands and the father's explosions. As they aged, the situation culminated with repeated admissions to skilled nursing for the mother due to physical woes and the realization that memory impairment was surfacing in the father.

The daughter moved them to a residence that was supposed to give both an opportunity to receive the level of care they needed. However, during the move, the stress of decisions about what to move, where to put things when unloading, and tensions caused the father to leave the apartment in a huff. He nearly knocked over a woman in the corridor who was using a walker. He went to a nearby hotel, paid for the night, and returned the following day. He was met by the administrator of that setting and security staff, deemed unsafe, and sent to a locked Alzheimer's unit in a nursing home.

I was asked to do an assessment and found him depressed and deeply saddened. Our residence offered an assisted level of care that was much more appropriate for him. At this point, he received medication to assist with his anger and depression, and the family soon found him much easier to relate to and communicate with. He moved to my building, and I worked intensively with him to help him cope with all the changes, to understand what had happened to him, why this had happened, to review his memory and other health issues, and to the degree possible, help him process the reality of his circumstances. The wife moved to the skilled nursing facility, then to assisted living, then back to skilled care in our sister residence, and continued to deal with her depression.

At one point, the wife decided that she really could not cope with the husband's memory loss, which had devastating and disorienting impacts on him. Standing by your partner through sickness and in health was a fundamental conviction for the husband, and his sense of purpose was deeply rocked. He had two strokes of a severe nature that caused him to go through months of rehab and recovery.

How do you unravel years and years of entanglements? How do you give yourself permission to let go, or see things in a new light or act in a different way? What is the karmic tie between these two individuals? The wife's depression caused a caving in on herself that made it very difficult for her to see beyond herself. The husband's attempts to follow the wife into her moods and make everything right or more tolerable had exhausted his ability to manage himself.

To what degree are we responsible for our own lives and our own happiness within a marriage? I have worked with hospice patients who are so ill that death is the only healing left that will allow them to move on and be free from the current trials and burdens of the body. Is dementia a healing, a freeing from a dispirited being?

....

Chapter 15

Alzheimer's as an Opportunity to Be Different

The Medicine Wheel

Oh GREAT SPIRIT
Earth, Water Wind And Sun
You Are INSIDE
And All Around Me

At one point in my life, I studied Native American history and legends, in particular, native views on education, the natural world, and the realm of spirit, especially those of the Lakota Sioux. As a result, I started running into references to the medicine wheel, or hoop, which represents the never-ending cycle of life. Plains Indian tribes such as the Lakota refer to the need to walk the medicine wheel during our lives. Doing so helps us understand different perspectives and embrace different aspects of ourselves and the natural world around us, as well as experience the sacredness of life.

In his award-winning book, *Honoring the Medicine: The Essential Guide to Native American Healing*, author Ken Cohen writes: "The four directions, or the four winds, not only help us know who we are but where we are. . . . Each of the four winds represents qualities that contribute to psychological and spiritual health, and a person who understands them is in harmony with the universe. . . . These concepts are central to all facets of Native American cultures."

The medicine wheel is still part of the primary orientation of these cultures and is used today in situations that need mediation, in tribal education, in healing rituals, as well as a navigational tool to assist with understanding the day-to-day events and meaning of life. This is a vast and deep approach, and I cannot do it justice in just a short chapter, but I find the concept of the medicine wheel useful when it comes to addressing issues of personality development and the shifts that occur with dementia.

In practice, we all naturally gravitate to a certain place on the medicine wheel, and in this way gain a deep appreciation of our personal attributes and talents balanced by an insight into our personal shortcomings. For example, in one situation, we may be quick to show initiative and jump in; yet, in another kind of situation, we may be too impulsive and not gather enough information before deciding on a course of action.

The wisdom of the medicine wheel lies in the way it helps us recognize our limited view of things, depending on where we are on the medicine wheel, and that another person's perspective, from a different place on the wheel, might give us additional insight into a matter. We then, hopefully, move in that direction, in order to understand a situation from the inside out. The phrase "Walking 10 miles in his moccasins" in essence means that we shift our perspective before passing judgment.

OTHER MODELS OF HUMAN PERSONALITY

There are many ways of analyzing life in order to understand what makes people do what they do, respond in certain ways that appear consistent, and find positions that work well together. The medicine wheel is just one model of the world that can help us view things differently.

Another model of human personality is the Enneagram, an approach to the psychology of self using nine personality types. It was developed in the early 20th century, but is drawn from ancient Sufi wisdom. The Enneagram was first introduced to the West by famed spiritual teacher Georges Ivanovich Gurdjieff (1866 1949), who used the system but didn't explain it conclusively. It was left to his student, P.D. Ouspensky, to write the first account of what he called "The Fourth Way Enneagram" in his 1947 book, *In Search of the Miraculous.*

The Jesuits found the Enneagram to be a useful tool for spiritual development. From there, it moved into popular culture as a result of the human potential movement in California in the late 1960s and '70s, when Claudio Naranjo, a Chilean psychiatrist and student of Fritz Perls, inventor of Gestalt Therapy, and Bolivian-born Oscar Ichazo, founder of the Arica School, developed the modern Enneagram of Personality. The Enneagram has some similarities to the medicine wheel and its ancient roots, and is a system that offers many insights to those who study it.

Other personality typing tools, used mostly in business circles, have not been around as long as the medicine wheel and the Enneagram, but enjoy some popularity. The Myers Briggs Type Indicator was developed during the Second World War, and was first published in 1962. It is based on the work of Sigmund Freud's pupil Carl Jung, specifically, his work with archetypes. The Predictive Index (PI) system, developed by Arnold S. Daniels in 1953–1954, was published for industry use in 1955 as an objective assessment technique based on assumptions of fundamental behavioral psychology. This tool is also used worldwide by numerous companies.

The Myers Briggs and PI systems help individuals and teams become aware of different ways of functioning, as well as how to apply this awareness to improve communication. These tools are also used to improve clarity with supervisory approaches and establish ways to help maximize strengths within an organization. Both assume

"The four directions, or the four winds, not only help us know who we are but where we are. . . . Each of the four winds represents qualities that contribute to psychological and spiritual health, and a person who understands them is in harmony with the universe. . . . These concepts are central to all facets of Native American cultures."

— Ken Cohen, *Honoring the Medicine: The Essential Guide to Native American Healing* that a person's "type" and way of reacting is fixed: once the original questions for both had been formulated, the responses given by participants created data that were sorted into statistical norms. Individuals tend to fall into certain categories, and even if it may not be the full picture, it is statistically enough of a picture to be quantified, analyzed, and conclusions drawn about predicted behavior. There is no expectation that reactions may vary—just better understanding of predicted behaviors.

GROWTH USING THE WHEEL

The medicine wheel and Enneagram models are different from other models. They assume that our development calls on us to grow into other ways of responding on the medicine wheel or the nine-pointed Enneagram diagram. These tools were honed over many lifetimes, through an oral tradition that added insights as it developed and was used in communal life.

American Indians have traditionally used the medicine wheel to attain harmony and balance with nature and events within themselves. By moving through the medicine wheel, they resonate with and feel the qualities of each of the four directions, and an individual can gain an understanding of which qualities are already strong and which need to be strengthened in a given situation, or in their life as a whole. All directions are considered positive and dwell within us. The practice of the medicine wheel is done daily.

To further illustrate this approach, I have drawn on information from the *Medicine Wheel Archetypes*, as designed by Andre de Zanger of the Creativity Institute in New York, and Ken Cohen's extraordinary book, *Honoring the Medicine*. According to Cohen, Plains Indian tribes, as well as individuals within those tribes, may have different experiences of the colors or some of the animals located on the medicine wheel, but the four directions and their attributes are generally described as follows:

EAST	SOUTH	WEST	NORTH
Morning	*Noon*	*Afternoon*	*Evening*
Spring	*Summer*	*Autumn*	*Winter*
Red	*Yellow*	*Black*	*White*
Earth	*Air*	*Water*	*Fire*
Eagle	*Deer*	*Bear*	*Buffalo*
Mouse	*Coyote*	*Thunderbird*	*Owl*

THE FOUR DIRECTIONS

What follows is specific information about each of the directions and how to work with them. Most people will resonate with one particular direction, but this is only considered a starting point in using the medicine wheel in daily life.

EAST

Quality: Vision
Animal: Eagle/Mouse
Season: Spring
Element: Earth
Color: Red
Time of Day: Dawn
Value Words: fresh view, be present, be ready for surprises,
all life is sacred, big picture, as well as immediate experiences,
options, and possibility

East Strengths

Visionary; sees the big picture; very idea-oriented, with focus on future thought and insight into the mission or purpose; strong spiritual awareness—attuned to "higher level"; likes to experiment and explore; appreciates a lot of information.

Overuse or Style Taken to Excess

Has the potential to lose focus on tasks; poor follow-through on projects; can develop a reputation for lack of dependability; can become easily overwhelmed; not time-bound, may lose track of time; tends to be highly enthusiastic early on, then burn out over the long haul.

How to Work With an East

Show appreciation and enthusiasm for ideas. Listen and be patient during idea generation; avoid critical judging of statement of ideas. Allow and support divergent thinking. Provide variety of tasks. Provide help and supervision check points on details and project follow-through.

SOUTH

Quality: Loving
Animal: Deer/Coyote
Season: Summer
Element: Air
Color: Yellow
Time of Day: Noon, Midday Sun
Value Words: heart, warmth, passion, breath of life, fruition, vulnerability,
humor, and forgiveness

South Strengths

An innocence and trust in others, based on vulnerability and openness; willingness to trust at face value; allows others to feel important in determining direction of what is happening; value-driven regarding all aspects of personal/professional life; uses relationships to accomplish tasks; arbitration is primary; supportive, nurturing team player; noncompetitive; focused on present moment; and intuition and feeling based.

Overuse or Style Taken to Excess
Trouble saying no; internalizes difficulty and assumes blame; prone to disappointment when relationship is seen as secondary to a task; easily taken advantage of; immersed in present, loses track of time; may not see long-range view; difficulty confronting; difficulty dealing with anger; may be manipulated by anger.

How to Work With a South
Remember "process"—pay attention to what is happening in the relationship between you right now, as this is of primary importance. Needs to feel decisions are ethically right—justify decision around values, ethics, the right thing to do. Appeal to relationship between you and this person, this person and others. Listen hard and allow the expression of feeling and intuition in logical arguments. Easily steamrolled, so be aware that this person may have a hard time saying no to you. Provide plenty of positive reassurance and likeability. Let the person know you like them personally.

WEST
Quality: Wisdom
Animal: Bear/ Thunderbird
Season: Autumn
Element: Water
Color: Black
Time of Day: Afternoon
Value Words: Introspection, dream life, release attachments,
accepting the shadow side, sacrifice, gratitude,
bless, purify, cleanse, maturity

West Strengths
Weighs all sides of issues; uses data analysis and logic to make decisions; seen as practical and thorough in task situations; careful; thoroughly examines people's needs in situations; introspective; self-analytical; helpful to others by providing planning and resources; moves methodically and follows procedures; works well with existing resources; gets the most out of what has been done in the past; skilled at finding fatal flaws in an idea or project.

Overuse or Style Taken to Excess
Can become stubborn and entrenched in position; can be indecisive; collect unnecessary data; mired in details ("analysis paralysis"); tendency toward watchfulness; can remain withdrawn, distanced; resists change and emotional pleas; may appear cold.

How to Work With a West
Allow plenty of time for decision making. Provide data—objective facts and figures the person can trust. Don't be put off by critical "no" statements. Minimize expression of emotions. Use logic when possible. Appeal to tradition, sense of history, and correct procedure.

NORTH

Quality: Strength

Animal: Buffalo/Owl

Season: Winter

Element: Fire

Color: White

Time of Day: Evening

Value Words: austerity, fortitude, balance, moderation, spiritual trials, renewal, deep germination between seasons, mental clarity

North Strengths

Assertive; active; decisive; likes to be in control of relationship and steer the course of events; quick to act; thinks in terms of bottom line; enjoys challenges, difficult situations, and people; courage; likes variety; likes leadership roles; perseveres; persistent; presses to get at hidden resistance; likes a quick pace.

Overuse or Style Taken to Excess

Gets defensive quickly; argues; loses patience; pushes for decision before its time, sometimes based on few facts; may go beyond limits; foolhardy actions; gets impulsive and disregards practical issues; not heedful of others' feelings; may be perceived as cold; may get overly autocratic, want their way, and ride roughshod over people and see things in terms of black and white; little tolerance for ambiguity.

How to Work With a North

Present your case quickly, clearly, and with enthusiastic confidence. Let them know how they will be involved and what the payoff is for them. Provide a "hero" or leadership role. Showcase, talk about the challenge of the task, provide plenty of autonomy, stick with established timelines, give positive public recognition, and use them in tasks requiring motivation, persuasion, and initiative.

THE MEDICINE WHEEL AND ALZHEIMER'S: DISINHIBITION

I have worked with some elders who have focused strongly on living life in a particular way. They gradually lose their inhibitions as the disease progresses and, for some, the behaviors exhibited appear to be the opposite of how they always were. This "disinhibition," as it is called clinically, can sometimes provide interesting shifts in interpersonal dynamics.

Some behaviors really do feel driven by chemical misfires in the brain. Neurons send confused signals, or parts of signals, and the individual exhibits aberrant behavior that is not socially appropriate or safe. If someone is stripping because they are confused, or hitting because they feel threatened, or being sexually inappropriate because they are triggered, these behaviors are not exploring some new aspect of themselves; instead, the person needs assistance with directing these energies and managing triggering situations more appropriately. These are examples of pure confusion.

In disinhibition, however, there is a shift in the person's responses or approach to things. For example, an introvert might suddenly shift to being an extrovert, or a critical person might become an accepting person. This is specifically what I have seen in some situations. It appears to be an opportunity for the person to experience another side of self that in normal circumstances would not have been supported before passing out of this life. It can feel like a balancer in the big picture. They are walking the medicine wheel.

In his work with the medicine wheel, Andre de Zanger describes the psychological qualities of different types in healthy individuals. I realize these descriptions were not being applied to persons with memory loss, but I see many parallels with how someone functions in various stages of dementia, and his suggestions about how to work with these types offer insights into approaches we can consider and use. In order to stay in relationship to the person who is experiencing changes due to their illness, we need as many tools as possible. Approaches like being positive and complementary, being quiet and really listening, letting yourself enjoy a spring/east moment with the one you care for when you are feeling more like winter/north yourself might be essential to your sense of success. All those moments of success string together and enable us to feel that we are successfully working with and staying connected to the person with memory loss, in terms of the big picture.

THE MEDICINE WHEEL AND ALZHEIMER'S: NORTH TO EAST TO SOUTH

I once worked with a niece and nephew caring for their aunt. This aunt had been very cool, critical, and self-important while they were young, and they described her as making "imperial visits" to the family home. After their parents and the aunt's husband passed on, being good kids they responsibly took on the aunt's care, but with great trepidation.

They knew there were problems, but they had no idea how severe they were because she had preserved social skills. On the phone, she tracked quite well for relatively brief conversations. When the nephew called to say he was coming out to move her and arranged the date and moving trucks, she was full of comments about packing and being ready and looking forward to seeing him. When he arrived, after driving three-quarters of a day to get to where she lived, she greeted him happily at the door, ushered him in, and all she had packed was one shoe box on the kitchen table. He had to call and cancel the truck, then made arrangements to stay for two weeks to get things organized.

He started finding expensive items hidden in tissues or tucked away in odd places, another clue of the depth of the general disarray. But sometimes such lessons take a while to learn. On the day they left, he asked her if she had her banking things gathered and she said she did, so off they drove. She brought her purse in the car and took it into gas stations. They made their way back to his hometown, where he had a friend working at the local bank. They stopped there and met with his friend, who usually handled only large accounts but was willing to be of assistance.

The nephew said, "Well, let's go over the account information from your bank and look at opening an account here." At this point, she proceeded to pull $81,000 in cash out of her purse. You can imagine the looks exchanged between the two friends and the nephew's horrified recollections of the drive and all the times the purse was nearly forgotten, the lengthy stays in the restrooms, and memories of her stashing patterns. This was the nephew's true initiation into his aunt's dementia and the realization that things were going to be really different from now on.

During her early decline, she was very much the same as she had always been—critical, demanding, and cool. But as the disease progressed, she started to change. She started to look forward to seeing her niece and nephew. She would pine for them when they did not come, and when she saw them she would embrace them, and eventually this led to clinging to them during the whole visit. This was very startling to them. They would stand frozen, not knowing if this was really happening or how to respond. I worked with the niece and nephew about relaxing and taking the opportunity to enjoy something they had never been able to do in the past.

The aunt became softer and more loving, and they ended up having a lovely interlude together. She continued on the path with her dementia, and they went through another rough period with her when she didn't realize she had lost her sense of balance and impulsively tried to walk. She passed away after multiple falls and complicated hip fractures. The niece and nephew looked back on the overall time they had together not as a burden but as a blessing. It was a time for healing of old attitudes, (North) sharing in new ways (East), and having an opportunity to just love one another (South).

"In order to stay in relationship to the person who is experiencing changes due to their illness, we need as many tools as possible. Approaches like being positive and complementary, being quiet and really listening, letting yourself enjoy a spring/east moment with the one you care for when you are feeling more like winter/north yourself might be essential to your sense of success. All those moments of success string together and enable us to feel that we are successfully working with and staying connected to the person with memory loss, in terms of the big picture."

— Author

THE MEDICINE WHEEL AND ALZHEIMER'S: WEST TO NORTH TO EAST

Another resident—let's call her M.—was petite, very proper, a well-educated woman with long white hair who had worked in a university library her entire career. She was a thoughtful, introspective person. Her family stated that she would only be interested in independent pursuits, that she would not join activities, and would not be particularly social. They also warned us that she would not want to pursue any religious activities because she was an atheist.

Initially, all these comments were true, but as she started shifting into longer-term memories rather than memories of recent years she started to relate to certain activities as a daughter in her parents' household, not as the independent woman she had become in her adult years. That young girl attended church, and she became very focused on when services would be and wanted to make sure she was there. She also started attending all the activities and socializing with everyone—visitors, children, other residents, and families.

The wing where M. lived had a room that provided space for activities and dining. Its windows faced a private courtyard, with residents' rooms opening onto it from all sides. At night, the residents' curtains were drawn, so no one ever bothered to close the large dining room blinds. One night, after everyone had gone to bed, M. came out wearing her beautiful green coat. She walked down the hall and stood in front of the windows. Soon she started this slow dance looking at her reflection. She began kicking up her legs and slowly flapping open her coat. She had nothing on underneath.

At first the staff was a little uncomfortable. Was this okay? Were they protecting her dignity if they "let" her do this? We had a long discussion about it. But she was doing it when no one else was around. She was showing some disinhibition by doing this naked dance, but still showing discretion by waiting until the other residents had gone to bed.

One of the difficulties of living in a supervised situation is not being able to have private, unobserved moments. Haven't we all danced at home with no clothes on at some point, or rushed around naked trying to get ready for something? We did this because in the privacy of our own home we could. "This is supposed to be their home," we say, but do we truly act on it? We decided this was something M. wanted to do, so M. should be able to do it. One of the areas of impact with Alzheimer's is that people become less able to initiate. This dancing was showing initiative, which also made us alert to some deeper desire or drive to which she was responding.

Another thing that anyone who has worked a lot with this disease becomes aware of is a sense of "This too shall pass." There are windows of opportunity when things converge or behaviors intensify. Staff and lay caregivers need to be alert to a sense of "What lives here, in this moment? What drives this? What needs to be channeled, supported, encouraged, or directed in safer or more constructive ways?" Within a very short time—a month, six months, a year—this ability, expression, aspect, or behavior won't be occurring. It will become the thing we miss about the person, even if the behavior itself was very challenging and difficult. It works this way because it was a way the person was still trying to show us something about themselves using the initiative that the disease continues to erode. There is a poignancy to this knowledge, which tends to soften one's tendency to judge or be critical about certain behaviors. This helps savvy staff to stay inspired as they try to find that middle way with folks who are having a rough time. How do you help them express other aspects of themselves when they are unfamiliar with these ways of expression? Why is it bubbling up now? Will it pass soon? In this field, some behaviors can be truly scary and dangerous. These must be addressed quickly and with a resolve to ensure the safety of everyone involved. But in situations where a behavior feels "unusual, or inconvenient," we may ask what is the deeper feeling or need that is trying to be expressed? And how do we find outlets for it while it is here?

In medicine wheel terms, I experienced M. as someone who had arrived in the West aspect of her life, as an elder functioning from the adult space and attitudes she had developed over her lifetime. It was predictable, as her children stated, but as the disease progressed, austere North burned through the mental clarity she had relied on for much of her life and removed some of the barriers to aspects of herself, so that the East, in all its freshness and simple joys, could come forth.

THE MEDICINE WHEEL AND ALZHEIMER'S: EAST TO SOUTH THROUGH WEST TO NORTH

My last example in this section is a woman who had been the family peacekeeper. C. had grown up as the middle child placating her impatient, gruff father and temperamental mother. She was the patient one, the kind one, the one with the great sense of humor and just the right touch with how to redirect a tense situation and make it better. This ability was well honed. However, she attracted a spouse like her father. They had a loving relationship, but her daughters would speak of her as a bridge mender, the one who would have to smooth things over.

C. had always been a polite, classy, and kind lady. The family moved her to our facility, and within a very short time a pattern began emerging. She would sit in the area of the hall that was the crossroads of the unit. She could see to the right, the entrance to the unit and the nurse's station, straight ahead to the entrance to the bathing area, and to the left, the dining/activity area and the exit to the courtyard. It was like the front porch of prime real estate in our world. There she took up her queenly throne (a seat by our fish tank) and proceeded to yell at people and tell them what she didn't like. She didn't like what they were wearing, how they walked, what they looked like, how they talked, what they were doing, and so on. She also tapped into old language that no one knew she knew, but unfortunately we all know: swearing. She swore like she had been raised next to a shipyard. This was absolutely shocking to her daughters, and they were very embarrassed.

We worked with this behavior in different ways. Staff would sit next to her and say, "Oh, why don't you tell me how you feel, but let's not let her know yet. . ." and she would direct her comments to staff in a normal tone of voice, "conspiring" and not escalating the other residents. To help get some of that energy channeled, we would have her lead bingo and shout out the numbers or help lead exercise circle, echoing each instruction the activity director made for the benefit of the group.

I asked the daughters how old their mother was, and they told me that she was 85 years old. I then asked them how long she had been the peacekeeper in the family, and they replied probably 80 of those years. My next question was, "Do you think it might be acceptable for her to have a couple of years of being the one who gets to express her anger, irritation, and annoyances, and let others take a turn at trying to sooth?"

She had been suited to the peacekeeper role, and it had served her, but she might have been curious about what it might be like to indulge her anger, to allow herself to lose control. This sort of thing isn't conscious, but Alzheimer's allows the loss of impulse control and inhibitions, and there will come a point when she won't be able to speak. This was her opportunity to go ahead and express these difficult things before she passed from this life. I thought we should let her have that chance to complete her experiences here, voicing all of herself. She continued to do this for about another six months and then it lessened. Once in a while you would hear a snarl and a snap, but overall it just gently calmed down.

In medicine wheel terms, East represented her ability to see the big picture and weigh future hopes against current strife and to hold her own feelings out of the picture and be an outstanding mediator for many years. With the disinhibition that accompanied the progression of the disease, she was finally able to experience the rise of feelings and passions and express fully some of these raw, unfiltered angry and hard aspects of herself. By channeling some of this in the facility and asking her to be in charge and tell us how to do things, we engaged the West aspect of the medicine wheel in her, which honors that we all have feelings and need to be heard and allows us to express ourselves. As she entered the North element of the medicine wheel during the final stages of the disease, she seemed much more at peace, steady in her mood and countenance.

LESSONS FROM THE MEDICINE WHEEL

The circle of life continues. Change occurs. Like the sun and moon, seasons appear and disappear—just in longer cycles. There are parts of our lives that feel like seasons and other parts of our lives that feel like a change took place in a moment. With this process, we are both the mouse looking at moment-to-moment needs or circumstances and the eagle flying far above it learning to keep our perspective and objectivity as a way to help us navigate the whole process.

The person with this disease also goes through a parallel journey. Short-term memory loss creates the energy of a mouse, the need to relate to what is in the present moment and in front of the person and their spirit; at the same time, though, the greater part of them is working on a much deeper and wider understanding, which may be difficult to see on a daily basis.

The reason I wanted to include this line of thinking in the book is to help illustrate that even dementia can be a season in the long life of an elder. Even though we may have functioned in certain ways in life, events can cause us to deepen our understanding of other aspects of ourselves that had previously not been revealed. The disease unearths that which has been just out of reach but available all along.

Chapter 16

Alzheimer's as a Way of Denying Change

Every morning for almost three years, E. would get out of bed, get dressed in her proper lady attire, and make her way to my office. "I need to go back to Champagne, Illinois. I have a house there, and although everyone has been very nice, and I enjoyed my stay, I need to go. I need to get my billfold and my suitcase from my son. Now, why my son has to have my billfold and suitcase . . . after all, he is a doctor you know? . . . Don't you think he could have his own suitcase? Anyway, I need to purchase my ticket, and I will be on my way. . ." If she then said, "Tomorrow," we were all in good shape; if she said, "Right now," we were in trouble.

My part of the script was to say, "Good morning, E. Wonderful to see you. How can I help you? Oh yes, I can call your son and get your billfold and suitcase. You know what I think we should do when we get the suitcase? I think we should wrap it up and give that old thing to your son for Christmas. He seems so attached to it. And then we can buy you a new suitcase." She would always laugh and say, "Oh, that's a marvelous idea," or "Yes, we should do that."

For plan A (" I need to leave tomorrow"), I would let her know that as soon as I heard from her son what time he was coming with her things, I would let her know and go ahead and purchase the train ticket for first thing in the morning. In the early days of this, I had to actually write out a train ticket for her, because she felt I was the ticket agent or concierge, so I kept an official-looking receipt pad to do this for her. She would then happily spend the rest of her day in activities, sharing meals with her peers, having basically a good day.

However, if she said she had to leave today, we all wished it were snowing. If she saw snow, she would ask, "Do you think it is better to wait?" And we would reply, "Oh yes, I think that would be prudent, or wise," making it her good idea. If it wasn't snowing, she would get very angry and want to leave immediately and feel we were keeping her prisoner and want her son to come right away. He was a busy doctor and, although he and his wife were wonderfully supportive, they couldn't always come over at every expression of dissatisfaction.

We struggled quite a bit with this. E. had been an independent, resourceful woman. She had two young boys when her husband died, and she raised them on her own, managed finances, and disciplined and inspired them to grow up into fine young men. She started doing stocks and other financial planning and became competent in this area, enabling her children to go to college. She was very proud of this accomplishment.

I finally figured it out. Although E. had been present when it was decided that she should sell her house and move to Colorado, she no longer remembered this, and it was horrifying to her to be reminded. She would be shocked and outraged and disbelieving and grieving all at once, and she would want to kill the messenger. So reality was no help in managing this situation.

However, if I said, "Okay, I will let your renters know that you will be arriving, but it would have been more considerate to give them 24 hours notice to clear out. . ." she would say, "Renters? What renters?" And I would say, "Because you stayed a little longer this time, visiting your sons and their families, and you decided to rent your house and make some money while you were gone." Then she would interrupt and ask, "How much money am I making?" And I would reply, "Twice as much as you're spending here"—or I would say a figure everyone had agreed to say if asked.

She would also ask to see the bill for her care. I had made copies that had one digit dropped off, so if her bill actually was $2,995, it looked like she was only getting charged $299 for the month, and for her sense of time, which was somewhere between 1945 and 1975, this was typically an acceptable amount to pay for a month's lodging with meals and other amenities.

She would ponder this for a while. Sometimes, she would tell me she was going to wait till the end of the month to go home, so not to tell the renters to move out yet, or she would say she still wanted to go but we should give them 24 hours. The next morning, we would do this all over again.

E. had a strong need to organize her day, to have a plan. This is called "agenda behavior." As with so many aspects of memory loss, there is a point when it is better to work with whatever the agenda is rather than get frustrated with it, fight it, or try to make the person find a new agenda. In E.'s case, every morning I got to see the Lady in Charge, the one who is on top of things. The rest of the day she was a follower, a participant in her own way, but this part of herself was not active in the same way the rest of the day. She woke up and united with the self she used to be and then caught up with the self she was now. Part of my role, responding from a place of kindness, was to let her have both.

Sometimes, there have been too many changes in a lifetime for an elder to manage making all the adjustments. Naomi Feil speaks about the "old-old" in her 1992 book, *V/F Validation: The Feil Method: How to Help Disoriented Old-Old* (republished in its 2012 third edition as *The Validation Breakthrough: Simple Techniques for Communicating with People with Alzheimer's and Other Dementias*), as a group of elders who cannot absorb this next new thing, whatever it may end up being, and live their lives in the context of that slightly distorted reality.

BC has mild dementia. Married for 69 years, now widowed without children, at 89 years old, she can't manage a world that her husband Earl is not in. She goes in and out of saying he is around or he is dead, or he had a sandwich with her, or is falling into the crack of her sofa bed as they sleep at night. We just go with whatever she is commenting and don't argue. She is so firmly entrenched in the reality of that relationship, and how it made her feel in the world with this loving partner, that her world has not changed. Everything else around her feels distorted, not the other way around.

It's very important to protect the fragility of a person who is doing this. They may feel quite determined in all their notions and vigorously defend them, but it is very easy to place a pin in their largesse and find a vaporous sense of self remaining. It is an important part of their coping to come at things with this belief. Let it be.

"Mother was an independent, reserved, strongly opinionated, and often critical woman. We moved her to Colorado once her memory became an issue. She always had her bags packed to return to Illinois and never forgot to ask about her return plane ticket home. Her personality changed with Alzheimer's disease. It was as if her inner child was released, and she became playful, positive, and fun-loving. She adored seeing children; her favorite restaurant became McDonalds, and we had to sit close to the play area to watch all the action. She was a great seamstress and created all her dresses. I became her shopper and would bring items from the department store for her selection. She loved everything I selected and wanted to keep it all. This response from a woman who returned almost every birthday and Christmas gift given to her over the previous 40 years. Our visits were generally fun times reminiscing about our family history, and she enjoyed photos and stories which featured her as the central character. Her response was often 'I did that!' In her dementia, her family was able to express their love and admiration for a mother, mother in law, and grandmother who had previously kept us all at arm's length. It felt good to give her hugs!"

— Ted, Son, and Debbie, Daughter in Law

Chapter 17

Alzheimer's as a Way to Let Others Go On to What Is Next For Them

One of the things about Alzheimer's that is so hard for family and friends to adjust to is the singular path it takes. The person they love is on a journey that will take them farther and farther away from the life they had created together, and from the ways they always communicated and shared. There will be glimmers and resonances but not days filled with familiar experiences. There is a progression, and those of us who surround the person work hard to find ways to stay connected and work with the individual in positive ways to draw their attention and focus.

There is a threshold at each stage, when the person is no longer able to manage certain aspects of this focus in the same way they had before, and it can no longer be drawn on. This causes repeated sorrow. We mourn each loss. Part of the reorientation process that the family of a person with memory loss makes is to allow and let go of their own expectations and, instead, enable what is to be and not drive themselves into paralyzing grief.

For many family members, this is excruciating. This is the area of the disease that is far more painful for those who love the person than for the person themselves. The person who has the disease is moving through stages, so they leave certain tensions, certain perspectives behind. In the early stages, they may have been keenly aware of how they used to be, and upset about not managing things at that same level of ability. However, as they move into a mid-stage level of progression, most individuals enter a phase of not comparing how they are managing to how they used to manage. They leave these comparisons behind in their day-to-day functioning, responding to the moment and how things feel. They display a straightforward approach to situations, which in some ways feels more detached or matter of fact. Sometimes, this is upsetting for caregivers.

Caregivers have at times been put through enormous emotional, financial, and physical stresses providing care for a loved one with memory loss. To have this person not respond with gratitude can be hard enough, but then to be ignored or not recognized can be maddening. The caregiver must let go of yet other expectations: to be appreciated, recognized as a connected person, as a primary person. Ouch! "After all this . . . after all I have done . . . after everything we have been through together . . . you can't say hello and my name? You can't stop as you are walking by and acknowledge me?"

I have heard family members or caregivers say, "Oh, he is ignoring me on purpose," or "She is so selfish and manipulative." It is none of these things in the perspective of the person with the difficulty. It is that their attention as a person with memory loss is now riveted moment to moment; they can't access these stores of memory experiences, pull up that particular file, the one where they have shared many common experiences with family members for which they should be grateful. They would be grateful if they were able—in the deepest parts of their heart, they are grateful. They probably cannot tell you that, though, unless they are having a lucid moment—and that may be occupied with asking about their situation and gleaning some insights.

I ask caregivers to ponder the person as if they did not have the disease, just for a moment, and to consider what the loved one would say to them if they could see the situation as a whole and talk to them about it. Most of the time, the responses I get are, "Yes, they would say I am probably doing too much, and they are sorry to put me through this," or "Thank you, and yes, they want me to take care of myself, too." Only occasionally do I get a comment like, "Oh, they would say I should be doing more," but this is usually based on the personality the person had prior to the illness and not the result of the disease process.

If we stay objective, we realize that the person with memory loss cannot help it, that they are unable to add up all the things their caregivers are doing for them. It shifts the focus from performing good deeds for personal ingratiation to one of performing good deeds because it is the right thing to do—the thanks comes from knowing that what the caregivers are doing is appreciated at a much deeper level, the level where it registers. In this way, caregivers can move beyond sentiment to a stronger, more solid sense of being in alignment and truly present. If we as caregivers bring our awareness to our time with our loved one, it will lighten the sense of burden.

A couple were brought by their children to tour our facility. The parents had a very loving relationship. The mother had Alzheimer's disease, and the father was caring for her. The concern was the father's exhaustion and his more frail physical health. The mother's need for constant reassurance and stimulus and direction was wearing him out. He perceived her clinginess—following him everywhere in the house, not managing if he was out of sight, and becoming very anxious—as a sign of love.

We knew this was a very common and normal stage to the illness, and although it was clear they loved each other, we felt this behavior was not proof of her love for him. When someone has memory loss, they often look to the active ego force of the one closest to them. Their feeling is: this person makes sense, so I am going to go where they go and do whatever they do, because they know what they are doing.

In dementia, displacement of a person's own directed sense of self is very normal, and the need to be in physical proximity is also understandable when someone's short-term memory is nonexistent. Object permanence no longer applies as it did in childhood (mother went around the corner; you can't see her, but she will come back). With memory loss, if someone disappears around a corner they no longer exist and this causes great anxiety.

With a great amount of encouragement, this caregiving husband decided to have her come to daycare for a period of time so that he could get some respite. She immediately transferred this behavior to others—whether it was residents she was sitting near for a period of time or staff members who assisted her, she would follow them. We stayed aware of when it was a good time to attract her focus to someone else, so as to not fatigue anyone. She also continued to respond to her spouse as a truly special person in her world, giving a little gasp of joy when she saw him.

She enjoyed being with others and many of the activities she participated in and coasted along quite content during the day, buoyed by each event. She was happy to see her spouse again, when it was time, but held no carry-over anxiety about where he had been and how much time had gone by or what he was doing. She was no longer able to focus that way, so in essence his timing in creating a structure for her that was engaging stimulating and at the same time relaxing for her was perfect. What he realized was that he had to rebuild his life independent of her. This became his struggle.

In dementia, displacement of a person's own directed sense of self is very normal, and the need to be in physical proximity is also understandable when someone's short-term memory is nonexistent. Object permanence no longer applies as it did in childhood (mother went around the corner; you can't see her, but she will come back). With memory loss, if someone disappears around a corner they no longer exist and this causes great anxiety.

Just as some children, in a fundamental part of their being, want to keep relying on Dad or Mom to keep running the show, there are couples who struggle with wanting to sustain the life they had together, but the circumstances of this illness cause one of them to take a separate path of dementia. The other takes on the caring and advocacy role and, at a certain point, also has to look ahead and begin practicing the life they will need to create for themselves as the partnership continues to change.

At that later time, the caregiver has to start drawing in the extended feelers they have used for their loved one, in order to rewire their nervous system and tune in to themselves. In essence, they are completely free to move in a direction that makes sense to them because the preferences, advice, or limitations of the other person on how their life was framed are no longer influences, unless they choose to incorporate them. This can be unnerving for some, and incredibly liberating for others.

Our model of marriage, as growing old together and caring for one another in sickness and in health, is being tested in our current times. I have seen families navigate this, with everyone loving each other solidly, being constant and true, and it is amazing to witness. It is a powerful testament to the strength that love brings to adversity—the ability to cohere not splinter, to have humor and appreciation not anger and bitterness, to endure with a kind of poignant patience rather then anticipatory, irritable grief. These situations are inspiring to behold, a blessing to treasure, and restore one's faith in humanity. If you are in one of these families, put this book down for a moment and go call or hug the closest family member to you and thank them for this extraordinary wealth of resource.

To stay functioning in this way, there has to be permission in the group to express what is difficult and to feel supported by others, even when opinions differ. The blessing is that everyone is trying as hard as they can, that this is uncharted territory for the group, and there is a vulnerability to this process. There is a spoken or unspoken agreement that an individual in the group can't come in too strong and heavy with their own notions or agenda, but needs to be respectful to where each person is in the group with this process. I see families do this over and over again. The functioning families far outnumber the ones challenged by old luggage. I see loving partners, loving children, pained by all this but doing a heroic job advocating, supporting, and navigating this process with their loved one.

Early in my nursing career, I cared for a woman with Late Stage dementia in a nursing facility. Her husband visited a few times each week, as did his girlfriend. This caused some confusion and consternation in the staff. I was repositioning the wife one day, and the husband was assisting me. We paused once we got her settled, and he began telling me their story.

He said he loved her so much, and there was nobody like her. They met in high school and raised three kids together, and they were happy in their retirement. But then she started having problems. She was a nurse, and she knew what was happening and what was coming. She told him he needed to get help caring for her when the time came, and to not resist that step.

She knew he was going to get depressed, and that he needed to think about himself, as well as her. That he was such a loving person that if he found someone else to share life with, even if she was still alive, that he should do that—that it would help him cope and be okay, and that ultimately she wanted him to be okay. If she died suddenly, and he mourned and was recovering, she would want him to be open to other relationships, if one came along.

To her it was the same thing, because part of her was leaving him, and although physically she might still be present, she knew the partner part of her would not be available to him. She was sure they would meet up again and work it all out, but to her it mattered more that he was happy in this life. His girlfriend was the nurse that she had hired early on to start showing up when her husband needed help. They had worked with her at home for a number of years and all got along, and when she moved to the facility the nurse/girlfriend moved in with him. This was a pretty liberal approach. I had watched the girlfriend interact with this woman, and she was gentle and loving and obviously respected and cared about her well-being. It was one of those moments of letting go of judgments that can come up with this illness. This can go another way. Because of the loving relationship the partners had with each other, when the person with dementia comes to a social setting, such as a daycare program or residency situation, they may seek out and be attracted to someone else, leaving the caregiver partner with some new dynamics to deal with.

W. moved into the memory care skilled unit after his last surgery. The recovery from anesthetics made him more confused, with agitated behavior, and his wife could no longer care for him at home. He was a brilliant, deeply religious, civic-minded individual. He was also a powerfully disruptive force at times. He would come into the activity circle and stand in the middle of the room and shout accusingly at everyone, as he turned his view from one person to the next. "This is the worst-run organization I have ever seen. Look at you people, just sitting around, doing nothing. Who is in charge here?"

I would come into the room at this point and say sheepishly "I am in charge here." He responded with a stream of remarks in a booming voice about my ineptitudes, and I would start moving toward my office, with him in pursuit. This got him out of the activity circle, so that the residents would stop cowering and go on with their day. Meanwhile, I would shift to being very sad and expressing how I didn't know what I was doing, and I had never done this kind of job before. W. would become sympathetic and, with his fatherly side, tell me all the things I could do to improve and what would be the most helpful approach. He'd pat me on the shoulder on the way out, satisfied that he had accomplished his mission.

W.'s wife was very faithful in visiting, working with us about approaches to use, and processing her feelings around the sudden changes that had occurred with surgery. He had a tendency to get cancerous polyps that his gastroenterologist felt needed to be removed, but with his age and mild confusion, she had been worried that this would change the course of his life. There were not as many options in that era, when it came to surgical procedures. Today, we see the use of conscious sedation, or spinal routes such as saddle blocks, and even the anesthesiologist making much more subtle adjustments during surgery with his own machines, which do not take the individual dementia diagnosis into as perilous recovery situations.

Working with certain medical specialties about the dementia piece and its impact on the total picture can be challenging. These professionals may really not know what problems come up with dementia. We sent a gentleman to the emergency room after another elder slammed a door on his hands, severing his finger tips to a degree. There was a small site of attachment on each one, and they were able to reattach and stitch them, but covered the area in a simple dressing and a laced splint.

The gentleman's main goal in life then became removing the splint and coverings. We would find him, to our horror, whacking his fingers against the table so that the tips were being dislodged! He had an altered sense of pain, which sometimes happens with this disease, so he was not getting a signal to his brain that this was not a good thing to be doing.

We jerry-rigged an ingenious contraption to help with this, consisting of a hanger bent over the top of his hand mounted on a ruler, taped to his hand and wrist, and covered with a cotton tube sock safety-pinned to his undershirt with another long sleeved shirt over it, and another tube sock pinned to it, and the whole thing taped. It would take him 40 minutes to get it all undone. This was enough time for us to attend to other needed things, or for him to eat, then we would secure it all again. In this way, his fingers healed. The staff at our local hospital emergency room had no idea what we were contending with when they sent him home to us.

When other health problems arise, there are sometimes difficult decisions to make, including whether or not to treat the person, based on where they are in their prognosis, the projected life span, and the comfort and quality of the life. It is a difficult decision for whoever has the medical power of attorney or guardianship, not knowing always what the person may have wanted to do in the past. It is useful to ask the question: Are we at a stage of curative care or palliative care? "Curative" means that if it can be fixed, healed, resolved, or held steady with certain treatments, should that be occurring? "Palliative" means supporting comfort and quality of life without doing invasive procedures, or putting someone through treatments they do not understand and may resist due to their confusion.

A recent example of this in my facility is a woman who has a chronic blood disease, which warrants blood transfusions every 10 days to prevent her from having severe anemia. She has a good quality of life currently and, although fatigued, is still doing most of the things she enjoys. The family met with the physician and as a group and chose to work with hospice support and not try to prolong physical treatments because of where she is in her stage of dementia. Hospice interaction is not intensive at this point, but they are getting to know her and the family and provide support; as things change, they will be more involved.

We had another gentleman whose prostate cancer was very slow moving, and the family did not treat this. However, when he developed skin cancer (he had been a surgeon, predominantly working with skin cancers), they chose to do the surgery and subsequent treatment. Although mildly confused at that point, because it was his area of specialty he understood what was happening, only needed gentle reminders to leave dressings alone to heal the areas, and participated fully in the treatment plan. There are no right or wrong answers when you first look at these challenging situations; it is a process of looking at all the options and weighing the most positive results for the person against the impact of the process, given their dementia.

In W.'s case, they performed the surgery because the risk of a bowel obstruction and the pain and problems that would cause seemed worse than the possible change in level of orientation post-surgery. He remained active for a couple more years. During this time, he developed a relationship with a woman on the unit whom he felt looked like his wife. In his sense of things, we could call her Marie, Marie 2, or "also Marie" as in Marie, too.

At first it was hard for his wife to visit and have him not wanting to leave the presence of his female friend. Initially, he would shift and go visit with his wife, but this got harder and harder. At that point, she was still taking him to restaurants and on short outings, and she wanted to continue to do this, so she asked if she could talk to the woman's family. They agreed that if Marie wanted to take her husband out, she could also take their mother along.

The wife shifted her visiting times to avoid alone time with her spouse and allow this friendship to coexist. W. was calmer and happier. She felt ultimately that he was living there, that she was a visitor, and that if he had a friend who helped him be happier about being there, then that should be a priority. She understood the disease would progress and that he or his friend may not be able to sustain this for long, and this was a more transient phase in their connection and life together. This gentleman had been a faithful mate. He still recognized his wife as his wife, but somehow in his confusion he felt this other person was also his wife. The wife, in her spaciousness, was able to work with it, validate it, and continue to stay in connection with W.

CAREGIVER SUPPORT

Many people would say that they would much rather have to deal with a sudden loss, grapple with the reality of that and the impact on their life, then move on to what is next.

With this disease, there is a period of time when the person remains in the physical, present in your reality but not in the same way. What that looks like in each family situation is unique. If you are the primary caregiver for the entire course of the illness, the concern of the Alzheimer's Association or any professional in this field will be: What kind of support are you getting? Is it from family members, friends, religious affiliations, or support groups? Are you utilizing some respite support services?

The length of time involved in the course of this disease, and the global changes that take place, are what lead to this concern about the impact on the caregiver. What are you doing for yourself to maintain a balance so that you are able to meet the mounting tasks of care with equanimity? How do you feed your need to have conversations, be spontaneous, and feel connected to hope and growth and life in its blessings, not just in its trials and challenges, in its decline and closures?

In the process of providing wonderful care for their loved one, caregivers may sacrifice themselves and pass away. Caregivers suffer more depression, become ill more often and, due to their immersion in the situation, often do not recognize when changes to their well-being are occurring because they are so focused on the person they care for.

Silver Linings

"Alzheimer's is a difficult disease that wreaks havoc on those affected and their families. However, as in everything, there can be silver linings. If my mom didn't have Alzheimer's, I would be missing out on being part of a community made up of other families going through their own Alzheimer's journeys. I wouldn't have met people who have had immeasurable influence on me and who will remain lifelong friends."

— LuAnn, Daughter

Questions for caregivers include: How do I adjust my energy? How do I plan for what is a chronic, rather than an acute situation? How do I expend my energy and draw from my own reserves in the long run? How is it different when I can't fix it? If it is going to go on for years, what do I need to do to stay in balance, to still be there providing care a year from now, or five or 10 years from now? How do I protect my nervous system, my immune system? How do I nourish myself? How do I stay fit during this time? What are my dreams? What are my hopes? What would I want to do if this were not my situation? Is there any piece of that I could incorporate that would help me not feel victimized by these circumstances?

One aspect in the progression of this illness that caregivers experience is that the person needs your support, your oversight, but during some phases of the illness doesn't need your engagement every moment. A welcome catnap may be possible while the person being cared for is happily engaged in sorting or raking, or safe sitting in a recliner or on a front porch, and they have passed the phase of wandering away. They are not in pain. They are not asking for something. They are peaceful. Such moments allow you to turn to yourself again—not in grief at the person's passing, because they are still with you, but in the type of companionship they now need, which allows time to probe the future and test what will lie ahead for you. To ask, "What will my life look like when I am not doing this?" This is the process of rehearsing all the sadness, the losses, and the scariness about this illness, and being able to get to a place that is on solid ground emotionally.

This is the value in having a plan of some kind. It helps you stay present in what you are doing, but it also allows you to look beyond the here and now. When kids enter adolescence, there is this annoying "rub" that goes on, as they test their parents' authority and their own independence. Part of that process is to start feeling like the nest really is too small for all this new activity, and that it might be nice to not have this stress. You love them but you start envisioning them taking their next step, away from home. A similar shift happens in caregiving, when your person is moving so far inward that it leaves you feeling clearly in a different place in relation to them. This space allows you to start looking ahead.

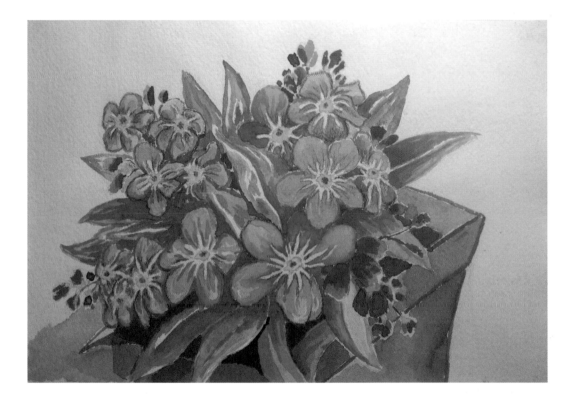

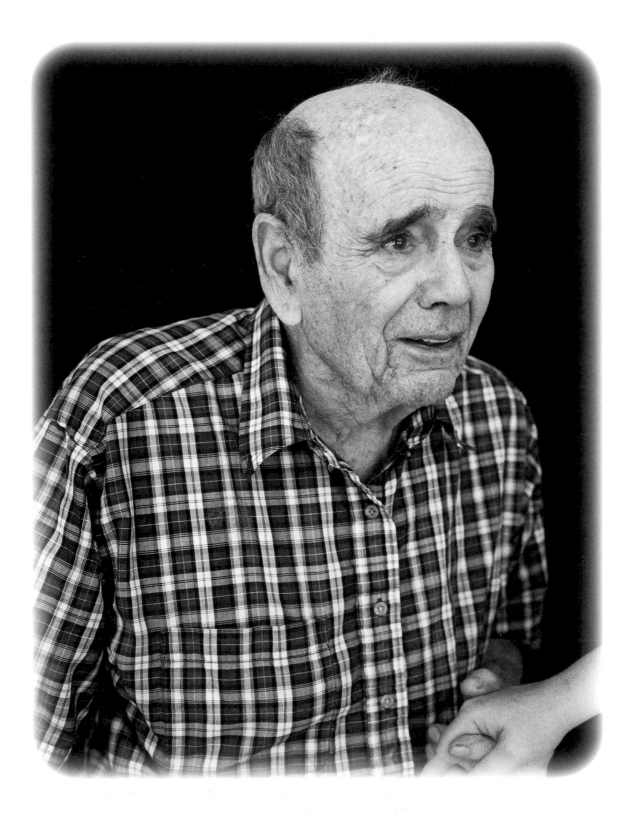

....

Chapter 18

Alzheimer's as a Path to Learn Compassion

The brain is a vehicle. It is not us. The mind functions. It is not us. What is the most "you" of your "you-ness"? What is the "me" of my "I-am-ness"? In the largest sense, what survives? What does not? What is shed? What is gained? This is one of the harder sections to write because from my experience of people's wholeness, even within the overlay of Alzheimer's, I strongly believe the work of the soul is continuing—that learning at very deep levels is occurring, and that these life experiences accompany the soul as it departs this life.

Some of us lead frenetic, fast-paced, busy lives, at a pace that is full steam ahead. Some of us lead purposely focused lives, filled with solitude and pragmatism. Some of us lead a life of service, whether it be to a job or a faith, our partners, our children, or other family members. Some of us lead lives disconnected from such webs, on our own thread, independent and not influenced by those norms. Whatever the life has been, Alzheimer's changes it. It slows certain things down. It changes one's ability to focus. It turns life review into a visceral recapitulation. We are not just reviewing our life in our thoughts, our brain and body are reviewing each developmental step we made in our life and physically shedding it. Yet at the same time, whoever the person has been, there is an essence that remains.

In many ways, the necessary transformation that a person with Alzheimer's undergoes is akin to being initiated into a new spiritual path. The basic existential need to find answers to the questions laid out above will cause some individuals to consciously choose to join a religious group or order to find those answers. Some individuals experiencing the dementia process may display strong similarities to individuals who consciously choose a faith-based contemplative path and enter a cloistered monastery or convent. They are having a similar experience, although the causation is very different.

Consider the scope of change required to do that. You lay down your worldly possessions and work really hard for a period of time on multiple mundane tasks. Your spiritual commitment takes you away from family and friends with whom you love to spend time, to a meditation center and into the company of the spiritual order. Once there, you have to stay really still for hours at a time in meditation, moving deep into the recollections of the past—sorting, forgiving, and letting go within the context of this present life, so that you feel completely resolved and at peace. You dispense with all mind-chatter and move into spaces in your meditation that you cannot articulate to others—places that make you feel so connected to the Divine that describing it doesn't matter. As we know, there are individuals who make this kind of commitment. It is less common in the current era, but it does still occur at different places around the world.

> "After one of my mother's angry rants, a hospice worker asked her, 'I see you are angry, and I wonder why?' She said, 'I am having a conversation with God, and people keep interrupting.' (Hands on a pretend wheel.) 'It's like I am driving along with four passengers in the car, and I'm trying to talk to the person in the front seat, and the two people in the backseat keep talking over us.'"
>
> — Linda, Daughter

I want you now to imagine that you are an elder with dementia and have had a longing to follow a spiritual path, but your life took other turns and required other tasks. While these all felt very good and normal to you, you still need this opportunity to feel complete. For some people, the silence of dementia may allow this. I have worked with individuals with dementia who have felt that they have moved into a deep place within and are working at another level in themselves without the mundane, the chatter. They are, in essence, "cloistered" by the experience of dementia.

Many elders with memory loss who move into this spiritual phase begin with the usual vigorous denial and ego-engaging will strategies. Later, around Middle Stage, that changes and the person appears blissfully serene. Illnesses resulting from anxiety melt away. Medication ceases for these maladies. The person no longer suffers from asthma, high blood pressure, and digestive disorders that were very physical and clinically documented—without the emotional stress triggered by their earlier coping methods, such problems disappear. They enter the present so fully that the cares and concerns that plagued them no longer have a handhold. A kind of gentle gratitude starts to manifest, along with appreciation for others in daily interactions. Wrinkles disappear, and aging seems to recede—the youthful countenance conveying the presence of a timeless aspect of this person. They are known to smile insistently. Sitting on their own, their face still reflects this baseline of harmony. When someone interacts with them, the smile broadens.

Family members will comment that this is the happiest they have ever seen their mother. Or that their father is so positive and just wants to hug them or hold their hand. Spouses sometimes experience this as well, but it tends to be a bit harder for a spouse. That's because of all the personal work they have to do to assimilate what is different in their own reality and their own expectations and losses. At times, though, I see spouses make that leap and enjoy the time they spend with this person, feeling their peacefulness and letting it soak in.

An elder in my facility has lived with us for six years. She initially wanted to leave and was convinced the highway to her home and spouse was right out there and that she needed to leave right now. A stroke had damaged her memory but her physical recovery went well, and she was active and capable with her daily abilities to dress, use the bathroom, shower, and so on. She had lost about 10 years of time, and during that decade her husband had died. We have worked to help her adjust and have outlets for her energy and to validate her emotions regarding the changes. She had lived on the East Coast and could not integrate the fact that she now lives in the western United States and her spouse was no longer alive.

Slowly, she has transitioned to needing more assistance, which she has started appreciating. We have begun seeing this constant smile. She tends to look up a lot, and there are some visual perception issues that we work with to help her walk or eat, but she is incredibly peaceful. Her son and his partner visit often and spend time with her, enjoying their time together. They are mindful that she is moving into a later stage and know that things will continue to change and that there may be some hard challenges ahead. But they are also aware of the spiritual quality that she emanates at this point. She is like a glowing angel resting in our reality. She has not made her transition yet, but there is something about her that feels as if she is fully accompanied on this side. When the time comes, there will be a release of the body but her spirit already lives in both places. We get the gift of that realm visiting us through her.

"It is said that Carl Jung would possibly regard the increase in dementia and autism as a compensatory function—balancing out the extreme we've found ourselves in, in our emphasis on linear thinking. The mind is loosening in a way that allows other faculties to manifest."

— Ellen, Geriatric Case Manager

"I am thinking of Barb, and how we developed a level of communication that was much deeper than merely words. She loved to lie in a recliner by the fireplace, snoozing. I would approach her gently, and settle my hands on her arm, or maybe behind a shoulder. She would smile, without opening her eyes, and I could see her body relax even more into the chair. As our massage continued, she often would reach over and stroked my arm with her hand. A natural reciprocation. And I would feel so nourished after those interactions, those "massage sessions." Something very genuine and loving was exchanged."

— Heather, Massage Therapist

Chapter 19

Alzheimer's as a Way to Teach Compassion and Introspection to Others

I want to spend a little time talking about facility-based care and the staff who are drawn to work in these settings, as well as highlighting some tips for caregivers working in a private home supporting an elder. Because of the opportunity to be in the daily presence of these elders and to be so closely involved with the daily challenges of care, there are tremendous opportunities for learning from the elders we serve. Many elders in memory care programs are master teachers—teachers who are passing along valuable lessons that are character building and strengthen integrity and compassion in their caregivers. In the intimacy of care, these elders shine a light on unfamiliar areas for the caregiver and provide opportunities for others to be of service. This is a gift, a sacrifice the person with Alzheimer's makes to allow others to be of assistance.

A person with memory loss becomes vulnerable, loses control, and no longer is able to direct situations, so the onus is on the caregiver to offer protection, guidance, and support. The caregiver must find within themselves that part that is able to practice lovingkindness, even during those times when there is no feedback or appreciation from the elder, perhaps even resistance and strife, and they must do so with a light touch in order to calmly stay the course. In effect, they must understand what it is to love unconditionally, and appreciate what it means to have daily opportunities to practice this. If a caregiver is able to feel this level of personal application of the skills they are honing at work, they will often begin applying it to other parts of their life. Their wider circle of those they love will be able to feel the lack of criticism and judgment, the lack of sweating the small stuff, and feel more loved and appreciated. It is an inspiring legacy elders with dementia leave us.

CAREGIVER TYPES

In the healthcare world, many types of individuals are drawn to this type of work. Some are on a journey through these settings, getting experience for something else, perhaps to become a physician, or a nurse, a social worker, or a psychologist. Some are looking for work that fits a schedule better with family life, the ages of their children, the work of a partner, or in combining their own education with family and parenting needs. Some are doing this kind of work because they have not had certain opportunities or education possibilities, and they can learn these skills in an entry-level position and find meaningful employment. Some are internationally diverse staff with advanced degrees, who are working on accreditation or on deepening their language skills, and they provide care as a means of doing this. Some discovered the role of caregiver and have come to love it; they know this is what they want to do to earn a living and plan to continue.

> "I value being around people with dementia as spiritual learning and believe that elders with dementia are spiritual teachers."
> — Ellen, Geriatric Case Manager

All of these groups can be useful resources within a team in a long-term care facility and offer rich and varied life experiences that elders can connect with. Sometimes, there are extraordinary and unique connections between individuals from very opposite life experiences; because they are in this shared environment, they are able to get to know and appreciate each other, something that would not have been possible outside this setting.

When we interview someone for this type of work, we need to feel their warmth. Do they smile easily? Are they calm? Can they give examples of their flexibility, their humor, their patience? Another staff person, who is not part of the interviewing group, might take them on a tour and have them interact with the elders, while the staff person observes for certain things and reports their experience. If elders can give you feedback, we make sure those individuals get the chance to meet and talk with the interviewee. If elders are unable to verbally give feedback, we observe their reactions to the person. Concern about how to teach someone to do specific tasks is not the initial focus; it is how this person feels to us, how they convey their intent or carry themselves, and how we feel being in their presence.

The residents pick up on the "messages" the person is actually broadcasting before they ever start doing something together. How receptive and open the new employee is makes all the difference in helping the elder feel confident or able to engage with the employee. You cannot teach kindness, or having a conscience, or being respectful—these are all qualities the individual must have if they are going to work with elders with memory loss.

Some caregivers derive their personal worth and reason to live from providing support for others. This ability to support others can be a wonderful thing in a caregiver's development, allowing them to move through experiences that lead to personal growth; by assisting someone else, they recognize their own contributions. However, if a caregiver is dependent on this feeling for their self-worth, it is a different dynamic, and finding the right balance can be tricky.

Still other caregivers seek approval, validation, and a sense of control over the person in their care through "helping them," and they tend to take the actions and behaviors of the person they are caring for very personally. Hopefully, with the right education and support, this type of caregiver can mature and develop the capacity to stand on their own two feet, rather than drawing emotional support from their charges. The other option is to encourage such a person to care only for elders who are not demented and who are able to clearly state their wishes and concerns, and on some level set boundaries in a healthy way because the caregiver is unable to do this. Such an elder would be able to say thank you and praise the caregiver's efforts and also give real corrective feedback should the need arise.

AVOIDING ABUSIVE CAREGIVERS

This second type of dynamic can lead to abuse in a caregiving setting, so if I pick up on this tendency in someone we are interviewing at our long-term care facility I am careful not to hire this person. If it is somehow exposed later, I make a point to make regular surprise visits when they are providing care. I watch them and listen to how they describe behaviors and what solutions they come up with.

As the daughter of a mother who was receiving 24-hour care in her home, I have had direct experience of this from the other side, as I mentioned earlier in the book. I was living far away from my mother when she had a severe stroke, and sometimes I could not get back to interview caregivers when a new person was hired.

On one occasion, I was immediately alarmed after observing and listening to a new employee—a veteran caregiver—expounding on all of her personal virtues: how she did this and that for Miss Rusty. Red flags were showing up for me. When she left her shift, I asked my mother what was going on with this person. She started to cry and said this woman would transfer her from the bed to the wheelchair with the Hoyer lift, which was our usual procedure, but would release it suddenly and slam her down in her wheelchair. My mother already had a crushed tailbone and took pain meds for this. She also liked to drink spring water, and we had it delivered to the house. My mother would ask for some of her water, and the caregiver would stare at her without verbal response, then go over and get water out of the faucet, while the jug was two feet from the sink.

This was enough for me, and I asked her not to return to work. I am grateful my mother could tell me what was going on, but she was totally dependent on this person

> "Since I first began working professionally with older people, in around 1996, I have been especially drawn to people with dementia. Usually, there's a relaxation about them (not everyone, though). Maybe because of the disinhibition, there's a direct honesty. They say what they mean. I find it relaxing to be around most people with dementia. Somehow, there's a lot less ego. Conversations are direct and in the moment. Even if there is a lot of repetition with one person, or loss of vocabulary with another, I have learned to drop my standard way of having a conversation. I have learned this from them. Instead, I follow what's underneath, which is very tangible. And I respond genuinely with words that fit the moment, but the communication is far less about what's said. It's all about genuine expression between us, from a deeper place. When I meet a person in this way, I don't feel that I'm talking down to them—and they feel understood."
>
> — Ellen, Geriatric Case Manager

while she was there on her shift. No trained eyes were around to observe good care or bad care. For someone with dementia, this is even more crucial. We are all familiar with the feeling of frustration and impatience, but to get some sort of pleasure from the victimization of someone in a disabled position is unconscionable.

BASIC ATTENDANCE

The opposite side of this is something called Basic Attendance. When I taught in the gerontology program at Naropa, a Buddhist university in Boulder, Colorado, they gave this name to the approach I have used for many years, and it is a meditation for me. Buddhist teachings underpin all of the programs at Naropa University. Programs that deal with contemplative psychology and counseling, religious studies, and the master's program in healthcare emphasize a deep understanding of what you weave into your perceptions, what becomes visible or available to you when you become aware of your own preoccupations and projections, and how to clear a space to perceive more fully what is presenting itself to you. Basic Attendance is being mindful while quieting the mind, releasing judgments, and allowing this space between you and the other person or situation to lead to insights you would normally be too distracted to recognize.

"There are so many stories. This work is just jammed full of potential for gemlike moments, isn't it? It's also challenging in the amount of presence it requires (not unlike children), but what a gift that is, really."

— Heather, Massage Therapist

I can find this place in myself over and over again in my work with elders. Being able to get there has become easier over the years, and the gift of this is to bring this ability to "stay present" into other moments that occur in our lives. Getting very still and just allowing is a remarkably spacious experience.

When I meet an elder with dementia, I suspend all of my preoccupations, all of my own agendas, and just become very present for the person in the moment—listening with all of myself and being ready and responsive, without expectations, to whatever may occur in our time together. The person with dementia immediately senses this and, if I can stay open, will show some availability in themselves to connect with me as well. Over and over, my work with individuals with dementia has forced me to listen in new and different ways. Because we cannot always rely on the normal methods of verbal communication, or what is being said is not the whole picture, I have to observe well. My observation may guide me, but my intuition also has to be engaged.

Intuition is the quiet inner voice. Many people are not used to interacting with this inner voice. For example, you may have strong moments in your life when you just know certain things, and you "trust your gut." In bigger situations in life this may be easier to act on—for instance, when you wonder, "Should I buy this house?" and all of you is saying YES, or all of you is saying NO, and then you make your decision. But in subtler situations, we sometimes deny our intuition or talk ourselves out of it because we dismiss these feelings as silly.

A researcher into the power of intuition in moments of decision, especially when there is a sense of danger, presented his work on an Oprah episode. As he showed, there is a tendency in some women to dismiss these feelings because of the social expectation that they be helpful and passive in many situations. This causes them to ignore inner alarms bells and continue their actions, but if they had heeded their inner feelings, these would have kept them safe. As a result, they experienced very negative events in their lives.

An example I remember was a woman who stated, "The house felt too dark when I drove up in my car." Her abusive ex, ignoring the restraining order against him, had broken into the house and was waiting for her. This is a dramatic example, but I want to emphasize that sometimes we "know" things that are helpful to us, yet we don't utilize this information because it isn't spoken out loud to us. Listen to your inner voice. Sometimes, the situation involved in caring for someone with dementia can be so trying that we feel at the end of our resources, but we always have our deeper knowing to tap into. Elders with memory loss make us go there on a regular basis.

> "If you remain open, there are so many gifts that are shared by these residents—trust, and so much more!"
>
> — Cathy Poole, Licensed Cosmetologist

I worked with one woman, A., for nine years. She followed me from one facility to another. She was challenging. She taught me a lot, and I loved her. Prior to coming to live in the first facility, where we met, she had been very high-strung and addicted to valium. She seemed to have had a nervous breakdown or meningitis, or some kind of insult to her brain, which led to amnesia as well as short-term memory loss. This was unusual in my experience. She was one of the more independent elders in that setting.

It seemed to me that when I got to know her husband that it was he who had needed the valium all those years. He was extremely volatile, small in stature, mean, and demanding. One of the things that irritated him greatly was for her afternoon snack to be a minute late. He would come up to the nurse's station and slam his cane on the desk and scream at us. I found this unbearable. I arranged with the kitchen to make sure her sandwich arrived early and would simply go and find them, wherever they were, 10 minutes before the hour struck, and this behavior would not occur. Another thing he loved to do with some innocent elder who had wandered into his wife's room in their wheelchair was to push them out of his wife's room at full speed, terrifying the person in the wheelchair.

As time went on I formed a solid relationship with A., and as her husband began to decline in his impulse control this manifested in striking her during his visits, if he was frustrated. We all felt this was not new in their relationship. We initiated supervised visits. Eventually he ended up coming to the same nursing care center, and A. was able to be with him as his illness progressed and he passed away.

You may wonder why I am telling you this story. It is to add a little needed background. When someone has an insult to their brain, it can result in brain irritability. They tend to be easily over-stimulated, and their emotions are harder for them to control. People in rehab for head trauma need periods of rest and quiet, periods where they focus on rehabilitation, followed by more rest. Sounds and visual stimuli are sometimes completely blocked out in a bedroom for someone newly injured. At times, A. would stand in her doorway facing the hallway and scream that she did not know where her room was. I would respond by turning her gently around and explain that this was her room and that she was in the right place. Her life history displayed a tendency to be histrionic. She tended to overreact in normal circumstances, and this combined with some memory loss as her brain injury was healing deepened her feelings of insecurity. This was topped off by poor impulse control.

Figuring out how to work with A.'s behavioral issues was challenging. She needed structure, and we needed to take steps to help her modify her behavior. I had to determine whether this was something I could ask her to handle as she healed, whether this emotional/mental health issue needed different support, or whether this was a part of dementia decline that needed to be accommodated and meant that we could not expect more of her.

I had this nagging sense that she was capable of more. I made sure that if I said I was going to be back to see her at a certain time that I always kept my promise. If she couldn't remember what was going to happen and when, it made her anxious, whether it was about medications or meals or activities. I was consistent. I worked with a calendar in her room to write important things down. She had done this before her illness and, within a year, she started marking her own calendar again. I would go to her room toward the end of my shift and chat a few minutes with her before she went to bed. We had a ritual of reviewing long-term memory events, then trying to see if we could pull up more recent memories, such as what the entertainment was today or what was for supper. Over time, she got better at this, too.

I talked to her about self-soothing approaches and what might be helpful to her when she needed to calm down. I felt she was over the top, and I challenged her to learn and use these tools. Sometimes this worked; sometimes it didn't. At times, A. would strike out and hit people when she was particularly wound up. If she did this to me, I would always remove myself without saying a word, then come back later when she was calmer. But she was getting better, so to me this behavior felt on some level self-indulgent.

I will never forget one particular incident, which took place toward the end of our first two and half years together. A. was hysterical. She had lifted a full-sized television from her roommate's night stand and tossed it on her own bed. She was yelling that this person did not belong there and needed to get out. The roommate, with whom she actually got along, wasn't in the room at the time, but in her mind, at that moment, she didn't want her to come back, as she was so lost in her own extremity. I was hopeful that we could figure out how to help her feel better about having a roommate.

When I came into the room, she clocked me with all her strength with a right hook. I had this moment of seeing stars and then this insight, "Stay and express honestly how this has made you feel." I sank to her bed and just started weeping. It really hurt, and I felt as if I had a few loose teeth, so it wasn't hard to have giant tears spilling down my face. Then everything shifted in the room. She stopped pacing and yelling, as if someone had slapped her. She suddenly fell down on the bed next to me and hugged me and apologized and demanded to have drugs to calm her down.

I just kept crying and wouldn't get up to get any medications for her. Then she got flustered again. I watched her mood and rational mind go this way and that, all within a few minutes. Then she dug deep and stopped. She got quiet, and she and I had a long conversation about our connection, my work to honor her trust, and my expectation that no matter how upset she was no one deserved to be hit like that. She agreed. In all the time I continued to work with her, she never hit anyone again.

Over the next few years she kept making little strides in her independence, her abilities to do things and care for herself. She loved the structure and routine of the memory unit she moved to and was able to have a private room. Later, the physical frailties of aging became more noticeable, but her mood state and behavior were very peaceful. In those final years it felt like she was finally in out of the rain. She was happy, and it was great to witness. It was hard to leave her when my career took me onto a different path. I met with her and explained what I would be doing. She wished me luck, gave me a hug, and told me, "It's okay! I'm ready to be on my own, and you'll visit."

> "These elders are giving gifts all the time in a profound way . . . it comes from a deep, relaxed, inherent generosity that is unobstructed and most often, unintentional, not personal, just flowing. Which makes it kind of outrageous in our conventional way of being."
>
> — Ellen, Geriatric Case Manager

When we work with individuals we really care about, insights will come. It may happen in dreams, in moments of introspection after an interaction, in a flash while we are in the midst of responding. At times I have dreams about elders I work with. In these dreams I have had meaningful conversations with individuals who have lost their ability to speak, or they show me something through their behavior that gives me a clue how to work with them when we next meet. I have had residents who have passed come and talk with me about their passing, and in one recent instance, asked me to give their daughter a message. This threw me, because I didn't know how that would be for the daughter. But I risked sharing the dream with her, and what her mother had said. It ended up being a very special moment for all of us.

When a new family calls me for a consultation, and to ask questions about this process, I begin to feel the person they are discussing. Because of years of being around the dementia journey and all the dear people I have known, there is an opening in me that tunes in at this point. It doesn't always happen, but most of the time I am able to rely on it.

One time, I read a book by a caregiver daughter, which she created from a journal she kept during her mother's illness. I appreciated her efforts, but it was clear that she did not understand what was happening to her mother. This had an interesting and disturbing effect on me. For example, in the early days of her mother's illness, the daughter couldn't figure out what was going on, but it was so obvious to me that I found myself getting agitated reading about the daughter's experiences. As the book continued, she described so many upsetting events that my highly tuned nervous system began carrying her mother in my consciousness, even though I knew she had passed. I quickly read to the end of the book, but that too was upsetting, because it was evident that the mother had not received best practice care.

I have to be careful about this; I need ways to unload. I was used to having a case load of 30–60 people, but when I served as a consultant for several years, my case load grew to about 250, all of them in widely scattered units in two states. Eventually, I found this way of working intolerable and chose to return to managing residents in one setting. I have found that I prefer this way of working, because it allows me to adequately address issues in my own backyard. When I was consulting and driving around visiting units, I had no control over the practical follow-up because the firm I worked for tended to prioritize our visits based on a number of considerations, not necessarily what I was specifically working toward on these units. Nor did I ever know how much support there would be in each of these buildings and the administration for the vision of care that I was suggesting. It started to bother me.

If I am being asked to be responsible for the daily existence of so many frail elders, my tendency is to take this personally. I know this about myself, and it becomes too much for me if I can't control enough aspects of that task to guarantee a successful outcome. My leadership strengths emerge when there is a specific focus, and I love being in one space where we can work together as a team and also develop our abilities, both as a group and as individuals. I love seeing staff grow in their work lives and in their outside lives as a result of working in a memory care setting when it is run well. I may eventually be able to manage a version of consulting on the wider outreach again, but only if I know there is really a daily commitment on the part of the staff that works in the setting to follow through on all the details needed to have a successful program.

The families of residents that we get to know are also part of our community. It is wonderful to see them feeling supported and their inner tension and angst reduced. As caregivers, we rely on the family history, and family members often tell us that they wish we had known their loved one before the illness, but they come to feel our appreciation of who their loved one is today. No matter how late in the disease process, we are able to find things we can connect to. This is startling to some families because of their perceptions of all the losses. This involves an active practice of unconditional love. An elder does not have to prove something, provide something, or do something that makes us appreciate them; they are just being and doing whatever it is, at whatever point in their process.

We understand poignantly how difficult this journey has been, and continues to be. We know that at times we will be tested in our patience and ability to provide care and support. Every now and then, a new staff member will come to us who has the impression that all elderly people are sweet. They quickly realize that we are dealing with meaty things, and that each elder has their own range of emotion, just like us. We allow and forgive when things don't go well, knowing the influence of the illness in those moments is not in the elder's control. We come back again and again to these two questions: How can we get this right? How can we work with this situation in a way that creates the most comfort for everyone involved but still attends to basic human needs?

When you work with elders with memory loss in this kind of setting, the key to success comes from recognizing how conditional we so often are in dealing with others in our lives, how rigid our expectations may be. We may need to bring more compassion and be more open to the flow and wishes and responses of those we love and interact with. The key lies with us. By coming from a grounded, centered place in ourselves, we remain who we are, from our best sense of self, even if someone else's behavior or actions is different or unexpected.

"Love is much more available to experience around people with dementia. Since they're less guarded, the human essence that we all have, of being a loving being, is very available if you simply sit down and interact. Maybe you're using words, and maybe you're just sitting with the person. It's like a very simple and easy game, to find each person's unique expression and style of being."
— Ellen, Geriatric Case Manager

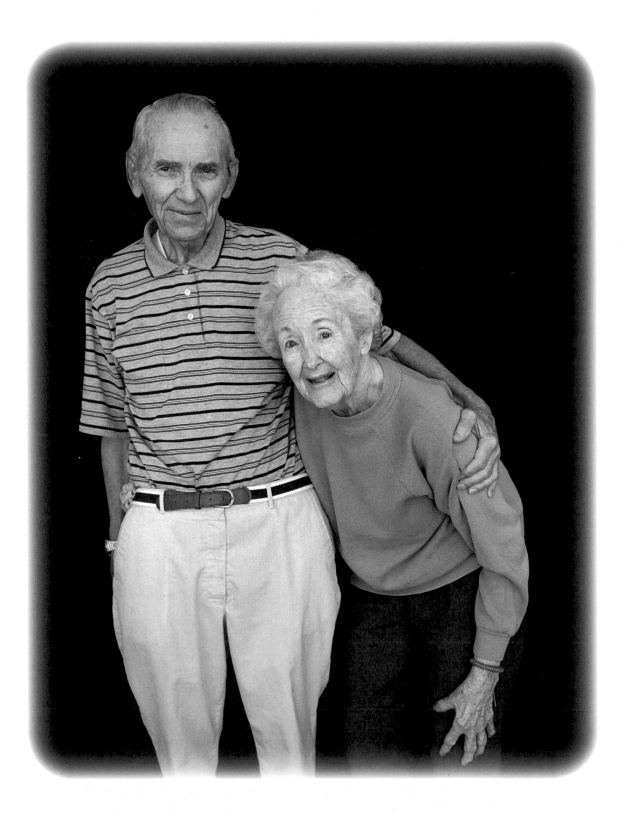

Chapter 20

....

Self-Care

The classic caregiver mode brings with it an intense focus on those people we are caring for, often at the expense of directing that same care toward ourselves. Indeed, I and many of my coworkers and families fit that category. It is my belief that we are all individually working on how to accomplish self-care, so the important thing is to support each other in that. There are many metaphors used to help us remember this, one example, "keeping our well full," replenishing ourselves to be able to keep providing the needed support. I have also used an image of a gas burner. This is a long-term illness that needs your caregiving energy over time. You can't crank it up and be filled with adrenaline or you will burn yourself out. You can't expend it all too early and sputter yourself out into nonexistence. For this project, you need a steady flame that will keep burning. Where do you get your fuel?

I recently did a consultation with a daughter and her father. Mom is still in early stage (Stage 1) dementia and very dependent on her husband. She is isolating, and wants her husband to isolate with her. For his part, he has a serious passion about anything to do with bicycles, and even looked into working in a bike shop after retiring. Because of his wife's anxiety, he has currently given this up and actually has his bike for sale. I emphasized to him that he is as important in this equation as his wife is, and that he will start resenting both the care he is giving and his wife if he does not keep doing the one thing that is rejuvenating for him. I told him that this is exactly the moment when the family needs to create the opportunity for him to get away—not six months or a year from now. He needs to get out and exert himself so that he can refuel. The caregiver is as important as the person who is needing the care.

Self-care is essential. If you don't take downtime, you will likely experience an erosion in your ability to be patient, present, and creative in your work with individuals with memory loss. They provide a mirror that reflects back to us how we are managing self-love. For each person, self-care will involve a unique combination of things that help balance the plus side of life against the draw on personal reserves that comes from caregiving work. It's a constant dance but worth every step. I practice everyday to be mindful and present to my own needs as well as the needs of those I care for, and the elders I work with keep me on task.

On our team, we have lunch-time knitters and folks who do laps around the building on their breaks. Personally, I love going to water aerobics, because it is social, fun, at times silly, and I get a great workout. Water also is very healing for me—the ablution aspect of being able to immerse and be out of gravity is immensely important to my ability to off-load. In my earlier years, I used to go for a run, but because of injuries I can't do that now. I also used to dance—African dance was extraordinary for getting inner stuff moved. Today, I take long walks with my dog, which allows nature to work its magic on me multiple times a day, not to mention the time I enjoy spending with him.

Many of us find being creative in some way refills the well, as my father did when he took up watercolor painting. Others of us find satisfaction and fulfillment in fellowship, such as faith communities, interest groups, support groups, or other types of gatherings. Still others recognize the need to do personal work, whether it be counseling, getting a massage or pedicure, or spending time with dear friends or family members. Giving yourself time for introspection can reduce the sense of overextension and lead to better work-life balance.

We may simply need to take a break. This can be a weekend filled with different types of activity, or a week away; at other times, we may need longer breaks. For family members, at a certain point, this will involve not providing direct care any longer and allowing others to take on that role. I suggest to them to think of it as sharing their loved one with others, rather than falling into a feeling of guilt about having reached their limit. This is a form of self-love, and at times it is the needed next step.

Self-care is essential. If you don't take downtime, you will likely experience an erosion in your ability to be patient, present, and creative in your work with individuals with memory loss. They provide a mirror that reflects back to us how we are managing self-love.

From one point of view, we might say that we are the ones who are learning and being helped in this situation, and through their sacrifices, the person with memory loss is making us a gift in order to assist us in our growth. We are being shown life skills that in few other circumstances could be honed so succinctly—to be persistent, to have fortitude, to be creative, to allow and let go; to value the impermanence of our lives in daily examples of the relentless change that someone with dementia is experiencing; to observe the bravery and courage employed each day, each moment, by elders with memory loss; to recognize our own fragilities and vulnerabilities; to grieve, to rejoice, to laugh, to be sad, as so many brief moments collect in our hearts.

What do we want from our lives? What do we need to make sure we accomplish or tell someone as we age? All of us will pass from this world, but when someone passes with dementia they have often touched many people as they journeyed through that process. We do not forget them and their contributions.

Chapter 21

The Importance of Humor

There is still a lot of life to live between a diagnosis of dementia and passing from this world. Amid all the seriousness, there is also humor. There are funny moments and situations that come up that at times can't be explained to others who are not in this situation. Other times, it is something that can be shared.

When I was first running a memory care secure unit in a nursing facility, we had an elder who loved taking walks outside. This particular day, the sprinklers came on while she was outside. She started running to get away from one, only to run into the next. Then some of us ran outside to help. She saw what we were trying to do, and she intentionally ran into more sprinklers, getting us soaked in the process. When we all managed to come inside, dripping wet, everyone was laughing, including our elder instigator. In that moment, humor was a humanitarian leveler. No one was young, no one was old, no one was ill, no one was well—we were just all soaking wet human beings having a good laugh.

Another elder in that setting was very little—a tiny person who loved to follow the path of the sun around the unit. Like Goldilocks, we would know where to find her based on what time of day it was and which bed she happened to be resting on: early morning the east side of the unit, mid-afternoon the south side, and late in the day the west side. She also had a tendency to fall asleep flat on her face on tables. We made a little pillow for her that she wore like a necklace, and we would slip it under her when we found her like this.

One evening, I was helping her to bed and we were in the bathroom. She had taken her shirt off and was looking in the mirror. She looked at me and said, "How old do you think I am?" I said, "I think, 90." With both hands, she grabbed her pendulous breasts, which rested on her waistline, lifting them up to where they "should" have been, and said, "No, I must be 800 years old," and laughed and laughed.

This same lady, later on in her progression, was sitting at a meal with others on the unit who needed more assistance. She was not very verbal at this point. She had a bowl of soup and found in it a particularly large piece of cabbage she had lifted to her mouth. She looked baffled at first, then she managed to make it flip. She paused, then turned to each person at the table and flipped them with this leaf of cabbage. This made others laugh at the table as well as her, after which she was able to get it into her mouth.

Many elders have had a great sense of humor their whole lives, and we see this mastery even late in the process. A look, a gesture will replace a punch line with just the same effect. Activities are a great place for humor to shine, allowing elements of spontaneity and whimsy.

Once, during the US Presidential elections, we wanted our residents to be able to participate. We all "voted" for the Presidential candidates by creating our own ballots. We are not able to send these in officially, of course, because in a memory care setting, the assumption is that folks are incompetent and can't legally participate in this activity. Some families continue to take family members out who can do this, but on this occasion in the building we did our own voting, followed the news, and watched the Presidential inauguration the following January.

On our ballots, we added questions such as: Do you want a knitting circle? A facility choir? A Spanish class? A facility dog? Of all these, a facility dog got a unanimous vote. We have pet visits all the time, but there was still a wish to have a dog.

In some facilities I had been in, staff shared the responsibilities of caring for facility animals, but other settings had not managed this well, so I opted to take on the responsibility. He is a Border Collie/Labrador mix and wears a "tux" in his coloring. He arrived in our lives from the Humane Society when he was four months old and has been a great addition. I picked the name Beethoven for a number of reasons, one being that it is a longer-term memory name that many of our elders can remember. We had the Humane Society come out once a week for three 10-week blocks to work on training Beethoven with the residents' involvement. There was much laughter and applause as he learned new things. Physical Therapy uses him to motivate elders to go on walks around the building. Activity staff will have him walk with them to gather folks for activities and do one-on-one visits with more reclusive elders.

When Beethoven reached his first birthday, the elders threw him a wonderful party. They wore animal hats of different types and made biscuits and wrapped toys for him. He learned quickly how to unwrap them, which ended my ability to leave presents out at the holidays. We had puzzle toys for him, which he figured out immediately, much to everyone's glee (some said he should have

Funny Things Mom Said

"I was pushing her wheelchair around the block, and she was singing a melody and 'doot dooting.' When I asked what song it was, she said, 'Oh, just the song we sing when we can't remember what we're singing.'

Once when I told Mom that I loved her, she asked, 'Really?' I responded, 'All day long.' To which she replied, without missing a beat, 'You got a little trouble at night?'

Once, driving Mom back to Cherrywood from my home, she was, once again, trying to locate herself in the world. She asked, 'Now where were we the other day when we couldn't figure out where we were?'"

— Celeste Niehaus, Daughter

been named Einstein, not Beethoven!). We have other parties in the building and a Fall Ball, with dressing up and a fantastic entertainer. Everyone dances and dances. Family, staff, and elders interweave, assisting, changing partners visiting together. It is truly a great time.

We also have a visiting therapeutic alpaca named Kaluah. Imagine napping and feeling some softness rub your cheek, awakening, and making eye contact with those beautiful big brown eyes with long eyelashes. Kaluah is comfortable going into every room and space in our building and greeting each person. He brings his head down and allows his neck to be hugged, and of course he is incredibly soft! He will even go in the beauty shop and visit someone under the dryer!

Children visit, too—either as groups from daycare, schools, or on an individual basis. Currently, we have an 11-year-old pianist volunteering who is extraordinarily talented. Kids come and help with craft projects, life stories, and reading. Our elders have an extensive garden program, with four master gardeners and two horticulturists working with us three seasons out of four. These elders are now in charge of making all of our holiday gifts for their families from things they have grown and made. They will harvest something and go to our kitchen and bestow their goods on our chefs, admonishing them to make sure they use it! The chefs will go out and let them know when a meal or snack used the items they grew. This is all accomplished with wonderful joviality.

Our daycare program is set up so that we have elder visitors who still are living at home but can attend our activity programs throughout the week at times that are beneficial to them and their family. Sometimes, in the beginning, this might be a respite break for the caregiver of just a couple of hours once or twice a week. For others, it might be eight hours, three times a week. Having peers and having a chance to be social is still important for elders, whether they have dementia or not. Initially, adjusting to a new environment can be a little anxiety-producing. The elder will be concerned about when their person is coming back or how long they are visiting for, but with support and encouragement we see individuals connect, make friends, and enjoy spending time in our programs. It adds variety and entertainment to their days. Although at the end of the day, they may not be able to say what went on, as it is for many of our folks, there is a fullness in their eyes. They have expended energy from using different aspects of themselves throughout the day, which we all need to do.

For caregivers who feel they are getting a little stuck, it can do wonders to bring some easy-access comedy into the space. We play "I love Lucy" episodes and other humorous films during downtime. Shows with vignettes that are funny on their own work well, and

"Example of one of my routinely enjoyable experiences at the community of elders with dementia I visit—walking in on a bingo game. Several tables of people sitting around with bingo cards in front of them, plus piles of colored poker chips. The activities director calling out numbers in a soothing, repetitive manner. At first, you may think the bingo players are kind of sleepy or not 'getting it.' But if you sit down, you cheer up. They are each carrying on with some theme—some may be flipping the chips across the table at the person across from them. Some may be busy filling the entire card with chips or stacks of chips. Some may be helping each other, even to cheat—and maybe not even know it's cheating. And so forth. But the main magic is that they're together in a suspended moment of relaxation and joining. What more could we want?"

— Ellen, Geriatric Case Manager

no one has to worry about following a storyline. We all must find ways to express the lighter side of things; it is an important element in the mix. When you lose your sense of humor, that's the quickest tip-off that you are in trouble and need some help, so do not ignore it. Look for opportunities to keep your sense of humor.

Humor is Contagious!

"On one occasion, several residents were doing various jobs needed to bake cookies. My mom was crushing graham crackers. I looked her in the eye, smiled real big, and said, 'You're doing a crumby job.' She frowned while she thought about it and then laughed out loud, repeating, 'This is a crumby job.' The staff member in charge caught on, turned to a man chopping nuts and said, 'Ray, this is just nuts.' He got it and giggled. Another man was shaping dough into balls. I told him, 'Things are pretty sticky around here!' Now others were enjoying the conversation and adding their own comments like, 'You're one sweet cookie!' and 'This is a cheesy job,' to the person blending softened cream cheese. Everyone laughed and teased for 20 minutes, and an hour later, when the cookies were served, those six residents were still grinning from ear to ear. One of them wanted to know when they could bake again!"

— LuAnn, Daughter

....

Chapter 22

When Does It End?

When does it end? I am asked this question all the time. I understand why it is asked, but my answer is usually unsatisfactory, because we don't know when it is going to end. Many factors converge that cause someone to depart or to stay. I have had family members get angry and rant and rage, "Why doesn't he just die? He's in essence dead already," or "She's gone! She's not the person we knew. Why doesn't she just quit and get it over with?" I have had family members still asking the question, "Is she going to get better?" in late Late Stage, when there are enormous losses in abilities and ways of functioning. I have had family members want CPR and every medical treatment performed, even though the person with memory loss is completely dependent on others for their physical care.

What all these family members have in common is that they are unable to let go of their loved one, even though it feels like the person with memory loss has been steadily preparing to make their transition. I have had residents stay alive to important birthday thresholds, or anniversary dates, or when family members come back from out of town.

In one dear family, the granddaughter had a very loving and primary relationship with her grandmother. She stepped up when her grandma needed more help, but the crisis occurred during the early part of a pregnancy and she had a miscarriage while trying to move the grandmother. With her grandmother settled in, she was able to conceive again, and during that time her grandmother started to fade. The grandmother stayed alive through the birth but departed soon after. Is it possible that the disease is influencing the moment of transition, or was it all coincidental?

I cared for one woman, J., who was a recognized master teacher in her field. She had been living in the Bahamas after retirement but was starting to wander and forget to eat, so her family moved her back to Colorado, where she had lived for part of her teaching career. She was multilingual and was truly Bohemian. She liked walking barefoot, could do any yoga posture, and when she would have her hair washed she would go find a spot in the sun and run her fingers through her long silver tendrils, saying in German, *"Langsam, langsam, langsam"* ("slowly, slowly, slowly"), as it would dry.

J. was a very independent person. Her daughter found articles concerning Alzheimer's in her mother's belongings when she had to move her, but this was never openly discussed. By the time she had moved back to Colorado, it was too late for these kinds of discussions, as J. was fully in her dementia by then. She would get up from her seat in the middle of an activity circle and approach different residents and try to teach French by saying, for example, *"eau, eau"* ("water, water"). Some would try to comply, and others were not her best pupils.

She and I had a magical connection. She had lived in our building for a while and was progressing on her dementia path. At times, her behaviors around dressing and bathing were challenging, but she was still walking well and able to spend lots of time outdoors, which she loved, and to eat her salads and fruit.

One day she fell, and it looked to us as though J. had probably broken her arm. Her family lived out of town, and she was able to walk, so I took her to urgent care. We spent time together in the waiting area, having our usual splendid rapport. The staff came and got us and said they were taking her in for x-rays. I asked if I could assist to help keep her calm, which they flippantly dismissed with the deft arrogance often only medical folks can convey.

Pretty soon, there was screaming heard from the x-ray area, as two technicians ran out of the room. J. had bitten one of them and scratched the other. They were very upset, wanting to know if she had ever tested positive for HIV. They wanted to give her a sedative. It was ridiculous and could all have been avoided. I convinced them to just let me go in with her and donned my protective apron, gave her a hug, put her arm in the right place, and they proceeded to get all the images they needed.

Afterwards, the MD came into the waiting area where we were sitting, and in her presence said to me, "You know, you can't ever let her walk again. She is going to have more falls, and she will have to be restrained in a wheelchair the rest of her life." I sputtered in disbelief, "This is her first fall. She has not been unsteady. We don't even know if she tripped, rather than it being a transition to Late Stage. There is plenty we can do to help her keep this skill and not jump to something that seems completely premature." I was very upset that he was saying this in front of her, and that he was issuing doctor's orders that were going to limit her quality of life unnecessarily. There was no discussion about negotiated risk.

She was wheeled back to my car, and we drove back to the facility in silence. I got a wheelchair and took her back to the wing, and she sat outside with a group of residents. J. ate an apple, and a staff member gave her a manicure. She was her usual self, no change. She hadn't tried to get up from the wheelchair, and she looked a little tired. One of the staff wheeled her in from the courtyard to the dining room, when she suddenly threw her head back, let out a long deep breath, and died. This was stunning. She may have had a fat embolism that had traveled to her heart or lungs after breaking her arm.

But I kept hearing the words "end of contract" in my head, over and over again—"end of contract."

J. had been such a radiant elder, a sensuous being, savoring simple pleasures. She was a master teacher in how she carried herself with this illness, she brought qualities of personhood to staff members who in some cases were struggling with how to validate their own lives. J. was absolutely present, even though she was not relating to time or reality in a traditional sense. She was relating purely in the moment and with all of herself that remained. If you weren't too distracted yourself to notice, it was amazing to experience. It was connecting to spirit, this vibrant essence housed in a petite, long-haired elder. It felt to me, that as long as she was fulfilling her role to teach us, to participate in her own experience in a way that included some basic things she still loved, she was willing to hang in and do this work of the soul. But if she could not remain connected to the earth, with that sense of freedom in movement and the simple pleasure that brought her, she was done. It was the end of her contract and time for her to move on, to transition to what was next for her.

I have seen a number of exits that seemed to be orchestrated to perfection. According to outside perspectives, the resident or elder is supposedly no longer present or aware, in too late a stage or too ill, to register what is transpiring. Examples include the resident who has been unresponsive for days, and the missing child or other important relative shows up in the room, says they are there, has time to say goodbye, and the elder passes. Or the "healthier" spouse passes suddenly, and within six weeks the cognitively impaired elder passes as well.

One of our elders, a dear, elegant lady who looked a lot like Audrey Hepburn, recently moved into a later stage. Very frail but still walking well, sustained by supplements and snacks she could roam with, she was a gentle, loving, and observant soul, even with severe speech impairment. One week, she looked unwell and suddenly seemed different, as if her vital forces had been knocked out of her. We couldn't pinpoint anything in particular, but she was not okay. We notified her son that we felt she was not doing well, and he said he needed to come in and discuss some things with us.

It transpired that in the same time frame that we had noticed a sudden change in the elder, the son had received his own sad news of a terminal cancer diagnosis. He began his struggle with radiation and chemo and surgery, and we watched her changing daily ("dwindling," as I have heard some older physicians call it). The elder with memory loss is hearing this voice inside their head, saying, "There is a disturbance in the field. I can be of more assistance to my son from the other side than I can be here. My son should have his life. I am ready to complete my life." It felt as if she was giving her last physical abilities in an energetic form to him for his use.

She lost her balance and did not try to stand again. She could not take in food, and we called him to let him know she was passing. He came in to sit with her and was shaking his head, "I was making the legal, financial arrangements to transition the responsibility of care for her after I was gone, and I got the news I was clear, in remission. They gave me six months to live, but I'm beating all the odds." She passed peacefully and gently, the consummate lady, at 5 a.m. the following morning.

I had a personal experience with this kind of dynamic when my mother was dying. During the many years of her illness, there were times when I arrived home in Pennsylvania to some crisis or issue of decline or just a problematic situation, and I would throw my

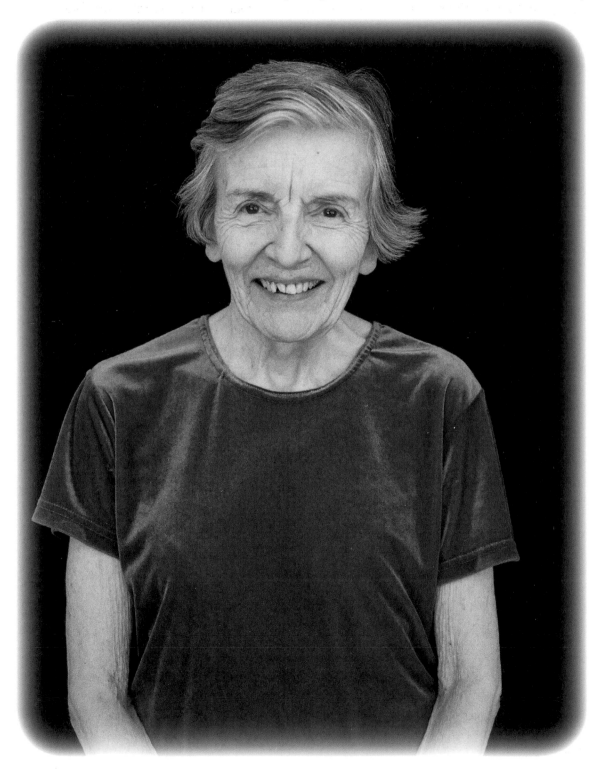

energy, resources, and knowledge at the problem and try to fix, adjust, or redirect whatever the situation was. We also really loved each other and had worked through all the stuff teens put their parents through when trying to define themselves. By now, we were very good friends. There wasn't anything in the way of that pure appreciation and fondness, except the tumult of all the physical extremes my mother had to suffer. Every time I was around, she would do better. She would be more energetic or brighter. She would eat better, sleep better, and things would just go better. I thought it was just because of what we were working on to make her situation or physical conditions improve. However, when she moved to Colorado to live with me, we learned how deep this all ran.

My mother had to have emergency gallbladder surgery. She had been taking a blood thinner since her stroke, so they had to wait 24 hours. I stayed with her, and it was enormously painful. The staff seemed unable to get this under control, and it was very hard to witness. Then surgery lasted much longer than it should have and because of it, she became septic through an infection in her blood. In intensive care, this caused her to have a heart attack while awake and talking with me and expressing everything she was feeling.

Nothing existed except that moment, with my husband at the time and an excellent physician as support in the space. The room disappeared. It was just she and I trying to get her through this very difficult, life-threatening moment. This had happened before, when she had had her leg amputated. She was coming out of the anesthetic, calling my name for help, crying that she was in excruciating pain. She was a very stoic lady, so this meant it was really bad, and I couldn't bear that. She had made it through those previous crises, but we were not going to see the same outcome.

This all happened on June 15. The building where I had just started working at the time, was in terrible shape. I had been brought in ahead of the changeover purchase, which was to occur on June 25, to assess what needed to be done and to begin working toward these goals. Mom continued her stay in the intensive care unit, and they kept trying to wean her off intravenous heart medication, but it wasn't working. Then, on June 28, I fell down the stairs in my home while getting ready for work and shattered my left foot. I was in the hospital overnight for surgery and was told I would need to use a wheelchair for two months, crutches with a boot for about six weeks, then just a boot for another four weeks, and would have to have a second surgery to remove all the hardware they had put in my foot. My older sister, Cathy, had flown in at the beginning of all this and was now going to come back to assist.

My mother called herself a dynamic idealist. She was a Leo who could throw her energy at something and rally. Even though she had been through so much in the past, she also had overcome a lot and continued to be alive and interested in life and wanting to contribute. She loved her family and friends, truly loved life, and in her mind she wasn't done yet. But it seemed her body was. This took a while for her to integrate and figure out.

My mother had a brilliant mind, with extrasensory perceptive abilities. Growing up with a psychic mother had its challenges, but it was mostly very positive and created what we call "plussages" in our family experiences. As I've earlier mentioned, I myself have certain intuitive sensitivities that assist me in my work. I seem able to tune in to people who have trouble communicating and to somehow understand them or the situation or the feelings and respond to them at that level, instead of always at the obvious or usual level of interaction.

I was having very active dreams during this period of my mother's illness. There was no separation between my mother and me—no distance of miles. I was always with her, and she was struggling with this issue of "Is this really my departure time, or should I try to overcome this?" In real life, we had to have a conversation in the intensive care unit about changing her core status. I had to explain to her that her heart was so enlarged and damaged, "boggy" from the sepsis, that they would not be able to physically do CPR on her. She understood and stated if they needed to use a ventilator for a short period they could, so we were able to openly discuss our options within the reality of the situation, but we were still trying to fathom its impact.

In my dream life, all this was still being processed. I was now in the worst physical pain I had known in my life, as well as in the worst emotional pain. I would dream that today Mom had decided to stop taking her meds, and that she was accepting of what was going on. I would relate this to my sister before she left for the hospital, and later she would report back in, "By the way, this is how Mom's doing. She's decided today that she will stop taking her meds." Then the next night I would dream that, no, Mom had changed her mind. She was going to overcome this, and she wanted the medications again; she just needed a little more time. I would then wake up and tell my sister, "Okay, today she is back on the track of wanting to struggle with this and live." Then, sure enough, Cathy would call from the hospital and say "Well, you were right again. She's taking her meds today."

I started having fevers, fainting spells, and incredible weakness on the days she decided she was going to fight this and stay, and on days she was letting go, I would not have any of these symptoms. We all started seeing a pattern, and it literally scared me, because I seemed to have no control over it. I realized I was lending her my vital forces, but also knew I could not follow her into death. This was a journey she had to make on her own. I didn't want her to go, which made it all the harder to stop this interchange at a level that seemed to be below conscious ability.

I spoke to my father about it and asked that he speak to our network of fellow Sabian students (the philosophical and spiritual study group my family belongs to) requesting that they put me in healing. In this fellowship, one has to request being placed in the healing focus of others. There is a fundamental respect for each person's process, resources, and privacy, and it is not up to someone else to decide I need to be prayed for or included in the healing ritual this group uses; it's up to me to let folks know. I knew what I had to do, and part of me did not want to do it, but the self-preserving part of me knew I had to stop this outpouring of energy—that Mom had to do what she needed to do, and I had to do what I needed to do, and that fundamentally we would both be okay. I knew she was transitioning, and I had to let go.

The healing statement was in a positive framing, "I am connecting to my resources. I am feeling whole in myself. I am receiving assistance in my own healing. My mother is connected to her own resources. She is whole in herself, and she is receiving the healing loving energy she needs. I am strong in my connection to my own life and all that I still need to do here." I repeatedly asked for divine assistance and thanked and appreciated this assistance.

I spent an entire night in this meditative state, somewhere between sleep and wakefulness, working very hard to lovingly disconnect the energy highway between us. In the morning, I knew it was done and knew she was now actively dying. We went to the hospital, and her situation had changed. We moved her to a hospice unit, and 10 hours later she passed. It was July 15.

We had had a month together, knowing we were working toward separation in this life. It was very stressful but also very rich, because we had moved through this time as a cohesive group in many ways. Ultimately, speech was crucial to my mother's ability to stay connected to this life after her stroke. She was still sharing her feelings and thoughts until the very last hours.

As I mentioned earlier, my mother had been a theater director in her earlier years, as well as a motivational public speaker about many topics and personal and spiritual growth pursuits. She had provided talks on the deeper meaning of the Wizard of Oz, for example, so when she departed, we dressed her in her blue gingham Dorothy Gale outfit, with her ruby slipper on her remaining foot. After sitting with her in the room for a while, we each kissed her goodbye so that the mortuary could come and remove her body.

When we got back to the house, an email was waiting for us from a good friend of my mother's who had some similar abilities to sense things beyond the normal levels of perception. In it, the friend wrote:

> *I think Rusty must have made her transition because*
> *I woke up hearing her voice. This is what she said.*
> *"I am making my transition now. My dear family has*
> *administered to me and let me go. The light and love I feel*
> *is indescribable. I am not in Kansas anymore.*
> *Remember, when you see things of the color yellow I am with you.*
> *I will be there to help those I love with their transitions.*
> *Remember, this is not goodbye."*

So it was amazing for us to hear that confirmation of the reference to Kansas. In the next couple of weeks, one of my three rose bushes bloomed again—not the red or pink one, only the yellow rose bush, just in time for her birthday on July 26.

I was unable to completely disconnect from her physically. For example, I "knew" when her body had been moved to the mortuary, then moved to another location for cremation. I "knew" the time she was cremated. I did the important work when I needed to, but there has still been some long-term healing, processing, and new revelations. Things have their own timing.

I have worked in both private-pay and Medicaid facilities. I have had residents who have lived a long time in a particular setting, then suddenly pass when family is discussing moving them to another area because of funding limitations, or family moves, or level of care changes. These discussions never occurred within hearing distance of the elder. Staff did not know or did not discuss it with the resident, yet the resident suddenly passed. Is this another contract situation?—"Okay, I will live in this odd and unique setting, but if it changes, I'm out of here." Why is it that others stay and stay and go through all the stages, all the changes? Is it just a strong constitution? Or is the project not done yet?

Those of us who work in the facility notice patterns in the transitions. Why do we have more deaths with a full moon, for example? Or why do they sometimes occur in threes? Does one person push open the door of the threshold, another slip through, and the last person firmly close the door again? What is the right timing for death? Why do people linger, when others leave quickly? I have worked with elders who say to me, "How can I help you? What can I do for you, because you are so helpful to me?" Every now and then, I will say, "What I would love is that when we are all finished with this life, we can get together in heaven and talk about what this was all about." They usually laugh but always say, "Oh, of course, dear," or "I would like to do that, too." I am still looking forward to this.

When I was younger, single, and still on that search for the right partner, invariably I would get into a conversation with an elder about their life and marriage and they would ask if I was married. Some of their reactions would be indignation, which was really fun. "What! A nice girl like you! What's the matter with those young men?" I would ask them for their prayers, "to help my angels flap the right guy in my direction!" Again, they would laugh and say they would.

I have had residents who have lived a long time in a particular setting, then suddenly pass when family is discussing moving them to another area because of funding limitations, or family moves, or level of care changes. These discussions never occurred within hearing distance of the elder. Staff did not know or did not discuss it with the resident, yet the resident suddenly passed. Is this another contract situation?—"Okay, I will live in this odd and unique setting, but if it changes, I'm out of here." Why is it that others stay and stay and go through all the stages, all the changes? Is it just a strong constitution? Or is the project not done yet?

So, many years later, how did I meet my husband? I was designing an Alzheimer's assisted living facility, and he was the owner's project manager for the construction. Even though I knew in our day-to-day interactions that these dear elders would forget what we talked about, when I married I knew they had not forgotten. Although my marital situation has since changed, I am still grateful for any support they lent me in fulfilling a dream, no matter how fleeting. When I struggle with a particularly difficult dementia situation, a behavior that is very challenging, or family dynamics that are very difficult, something that feels like a knot, I ask all the folks I have worked with before, who have died, and who are still interested in this dementia experience, if they could lend their understanding and compassion to us and help us with our situation.

The first national Alzheimer's conference that I attended was in Chicago in 1991. The organizers had expected 500 participants; 1,000 people showed up from all over the country—researchers, educators, professional and lay caregivers, and family members gathered in one gigantic room. When the first thunderous applause broke out, I burst into tears. I could sense there was a matching applause and feeling of excitement from our invisible attendees. I could hear their voices saying, "Finally, finally, you have all come together! Now the work really begins! Hurray! Hurray!"

People who had died from the disease, or had worked with it in their own families, or who had thought seriously about it related to research or professionally, were part of a great stream of consciousness working on this "Dementia Project." Those of us physically in the room were stepping up to take the baton on its next leg of the journey. Depending on our individual gifts and talents, we will make progress with the disease and its impacts. Individually, this might manifest as becoming more aware, being more real about life and its challenges. It might manifest as improving quality of life or finding a cure. It is all part of a flow of effort, and I feel deeply connected to this stream of work.

It amazes me that we as human beings can choose from so many different endeavors in life in order to find what we are passionate about, and that progress that can be made when we come together in a shared mission. Someone starts it, someone joins in, someone takes over, the players change, but the contributions continue year after year, century after century.

The arts, the sciences, sports—our human impulse to improve something, no matter how limited our perspective, is manifested in multiple ways. Sometimes, in hindsight, we realize it wasn't an improvement and then we have to try again. In spiritual teachings, this is called "the evolution of man," this reaching toward the spirit, directionally upward. And we need to be aware that the spirit works involutionally toward man, or from above toward humanity.

Symbols of this idea can be traced from ancient to modern times. Examples include the stations of the Tree of Life in their increasing complexity and nuance as one ascends the image, in Judaic cabalistic drawings; the dove, the hand of God, and other images coming from the clouds, appearing in Christian art; or the kundalini serpent that rises in the spine of man with spiritual awakening in the Hindu faith. What is it in us that continually aspires? And how tragic and lost we are when we lose track of this part of ourself. What makes a child keep trying to walk, when in the beginning that head is so big and wobbly and those little legs so ungainly and the cushion of the diaper so appreciated? Somehow, even in that little example, we see this fundamental birthright instinctively in action.

Chapter 23

....

Conclusion

My hope is that we will be able to find a cure for Alzheimer's and that elders with dementia and Alzheimer's will have access to the best support and care possible as they experience their progression. I hope we will move away from ageism and dementia-ism, and that we will recognize that as we age we are all timeless beings within our physical packages.

Oriented elders know this. If you ask them how old they feel inwardly, most will say, "Somewhere between 35 and 45" (this statement may even come from the lips of an elder in their 90s). Even though the physical has its realities, a parallel experience is going on inside that does not relate on some level to the aging exterior. We are not our packages; they are an expression of us, a vehicle to use in this lifetime, but not the sole definition of who we are.

My aging brain is part of my physical experience during my journey on the planet in this lifetime. But where do my memories rest? Do they belong to the matter of the brain, or to my spirit? If I can't draw them forth to share with others, does that mean they are gone? Or does it simply mean the retrieval system in my file bank has been broken, and my ability to express them impaired?

Who is the person who has continued to change throughout their lifetime in such strong phases that many aspects of these episodes cannot be remembered? Do we react in shock when someone can't remember the first two, three, or five years of their life? We know that all of those early experiences were registered and used to develop and function in the world, so why are we so hard on elders when their memory falters in what may be the last three to five years of their lives? Why do we say things like, "They are already dead," or "That's not my father"? I think we come together for very specific reasons and that we have things to learn from each other. No matter how great or hard something is, it is all part of the same package of human life.

What meaning do you want your life to have? What do you want to resolve, to learn, to forgive? What do you want to make sure you accomplish before your passing? How can you hone your life skills to build character, honesty, patience, fortitude, persistence, positive approaches to life, to be kind, loving, and compassionate? People with memory loss facilitate that process in everyone they come into contact with. And they do it in really concrete ways, with no pussy-footing around. That is an amazing contribution to all of us.

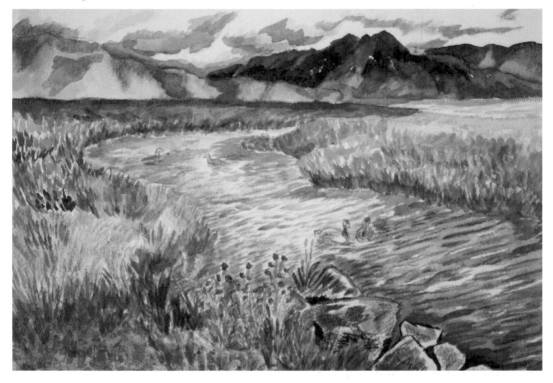

If you are still alive, you are still learning, still contributing, and still productive in your own unique way in our human community. At times, humans are extraordinarily judgmental about what they view as constructive or contributing. People with memory loss are trying as hard as they can. In the face of something daunting they show courage, bravery, dignity, love, and humor. They are living reminders to those they meet about the importance of going deeper.

What meaning do you want your life to have? What do you want to resolve, to learn, to forgive? What do you want to make sure you accomplish before your passing? How can you hone your life skills to build character, honesty, patience, fortitude, persistence, positive approaches to life, to be kind, loving, and compassionate? People with memory loss facilitate that process in everyone they come into contact with. And they do it in really concrete ways, with no pussy-footing around. That is an amazing contribution to all of us.

I believe we each have an essence—a beautiful, loving, completely whole and well inner aspect of our being. This is united with all the joy, love, and goodness of a creative universal force. It does not disappear because of a brain illness. It does not disappear because of death. On a deep soul level, all of these experiences are registering in ways only that soul will know and utilize in its greater becoming.

Best wishes on your journey,
Megan

Appreciation and Gratitude

I would like to thank the following people:

My parents, Rusty and Stan Carnarius, for their wonderful parenting, their brilliance of mind, mature humanity, and their deep belief in Spirit, and for allowing me to grow up as an individual and a creative thinker. Special thanks to my father, Stan, for his merciful editing and clarity, helping this project get to the finish line.

My siblings—Cathy, for her big-sister leadership, innate sense of systems, and how to get things done, even with this project; Becky, for her humor and the things she has taught me about looking deeper.

My grandparents, and great grandmothers, for aging as gracefully as fine wine, for being vivid teachers, and making me want you to be proud.

Dr. Henry Williams, an extraordinary medical practitioner! Ursel Peitzner, for her wisdom and mentoring during my years in Camphill. Fredy and Mimi Buchwalder, for teaching me about alternative lifestyles and living as artist. Marilyn Israel, for believing in my abilities and giving me career opportunities to express my passion.

Elisabeth Borden, a precious colleague, pushing me to the next level with job skills, for the award-winning design experience. Naropa University, for my adjunct faculty role for five years, working with wonderful students in the gerontology masters program. Richard, for your initial technical support, and Lindsay your technical help at the end. Emily Snyder for your graphic artist skills. The Dog Spot in Boulder, and Karrla and family for helping with Beethoven. Liza Weems for your beautiful skills with photography.

A big thank you, too, to my wonderful team, employer, co-workers, and friends, residents, and families at Balfour Cherrywood Village and the sister residences of Balfour Senior Living.

Thank you for growing up in The Society of Friends (Quakers) and for the belief "that each of us has that of God within us" and "the spirit moves each person in their own way"; for the foundation of the Sabian work, by Marc Edmund Jones and Sabian Assembly, through which many insights have been fueled in our family, and whose fellowship brought more exposure to wise and beloved elders.

Thank you, Nicky Leach, for your extraordinary editing skills and patience teaching me about this process. Thank you, Thierry Bogliolo and Sabine Weeke, for making this dream a reality, and everyone at Findhorn Press—Carol Shaw, Mieke Wik, Gail Torr, Elaine Harrison, Richard Crookes and Joan Pinkert for orchestrating the raw materials into this beautiful offering and getting it out into the world.

We would like to thank all contributors to this book for sharing their quotes and stories with us. We gratefully acknowledge permission to use this material within the context of the book. This includes the following: LuAnn Gourley; Ted and Debbie Appel; Jeff Weltzin; Celeste M. Niehaus; Linda Whitney; KAD; Laurel Alterman; B. Valerie Peckler; Bobbi LaPlaca; Victor Hoerner; Betty Armantrout; Diane Lawrence; Phyllis Olivas; Judy Dickinson; Heather Grimes; Ellen Knapp, MA, LFC, Geriatric Case Manager; Karrla McGee; Cathy Poole; and Amanda McCracken.

Thank you to the Alzheimer's Association, for all the education and opportunities to be of service. I want to give a special callout to the 14 years that I spent on the education committee, working with a wonderfully inspiring group of dedicated professionals.

I also want to thank the families and individuals with Alzheimer's disease and other dementias I have worked with, and the insights they have given me and continue to provide. Thank you for the opportunities for humbling mistakes, piercing life lessons, witnessing examples of fortitude and enduring love. Thank you most of all for the chance to be in the presence of these brave individuals.

Appendix

A Little History and Guidance on
Medications for Behaviors

In the best-case scenario, we live into our elder years in good health, not needing to take any prescription or over-the-counter medications or supplements. But if these are indicated, the next best-case scenario is for the necessary medications and or/helpful supplements to be tracked and supervised in a coordinated way to ensure that the senior stays in the best health for their condition.

Best practices regarding medications and seniors revolve around some important concepts. The first is that medications interact with one another and must be monitored. At times, a person may be seeing different doctors and not realize they should be notifying each of them about every medication and/or supplement they are taking.

THE RULE OF SIX

The pharmaceutical world promotes the idea of the Rule of Six, to encourage medication evaluation in individuals over the age of 65 to assess if the total number of drugs they are taking can be reduced to six or less. For example, in some instances, an individual may be taking two drugs for the same medical condition and may be able to eliminate one of them; similarly, the different actions of a single drug may mean that it can be taken to manage two separate medical conditions, thereby cutting down on medications.

When a person has multiple diagnosed medical conditions, all of which need different specific medications, no matter what one tries to do to reduce the number of medications, it may be medically necessary to take them all. In this type of situation, it's important to periodically review the medications to see if the problem still exists after the person has developed dementia, because sometimes illnesses are psychosomatic in origin. One example is hypertension, which can result from lifestyle choices, as well as genetic factors. Medication for hypertension may be able to be discontinued if, for example, the person is no longer in a stressful job or living situation or their memory loss means that stressful thought patterns are no longer present in their awareness. They may have also moved into a restless stage of dementia, leading to them losing the weight that had once created the need for medication. Asthma can be the same way. We have had certain individuals stop all asthma medication once far enough into the progression, because attacks simply stop.

COMPLEMENTARY MEDICINE

Some families work with complementary medicine options for their elder members, and normally know and trust the practitioner enough to ask for a consultation. At the facility in Colorado where I work, complementary therapies used by families include Bach flower remedies, homeopathy, aromatherapy, massage therapy, chiropractic services, music therapy, speech therapy, cognitive therapies, acupuncture, herbal tinctures and supplements, and nutritional changes such as limiting caffeine and sugar and switching to a gluten-free diet.

The challenge for those families with loved ones living in residential settings who want to use such approaches is that they must first seek approval of the primary physician, who will then provide doctor's orders under their own license for use of alternative medical approaches in the facility. When the MD is familiar with the modality and is supportive of the family and their efforts, this type of approval is possible; if, however, the MD is unfamiliar with the modality, he or she will often refuse to provide the necessary doctor's orders so it can be used, which effectively ties the hands of the family in pursuing this option for their elder in the facility. If the person is mobile and can handle going out for alternative treatments, that can work for a time, but the staff in the building cannot administer any remedies, whether internal or topical, without the necessary doctor's orders to do so. Of course, if the individual still lives at home, family caregivers and friends may be able to provide these options for as long as they are effective.

If the person with memory loss progresses past the particular health concern and no longer needs complementary treatments, they can be stopped. More commonly, at a certain point in dementia progression, alternative approaches to treatment cannot access the changes in the brain deeply enough, so they no longer work.

Another issue is that sometimes the person with dementia is no longer able to understand the importance of taking or experiencing these remedies and treatments and begins refusing or simply cannot manage what is required of them to participate. Although we all wish these alternative approaches could still help them, sometimes we have to move into allopathic pharmaceuticals to help with the stress and or safety concerns the behaviors are causing.

MEDICATION GUIDELINES FOR SENIORS

Early in drug-testing phases, when new drugs are being prepared for approval by the FDA prior to release, pharmaceutical companies use volunteers to test the drugs. These volunteers have tended to be young, typically under the age of 35, and in good health. The Beers Criteria for Inappropriate Medication Use in Older Adults is a standard that was developed in response to poor medication reactions to certain types of medications in some seniors. For this list, additional research was done specifically on seniors.

In monitoring the adverse effects some medications can have on seniors, researchers noted that this was due to common physiological changes in aging bodies. Seniors have a tendency to have less acidity in their gastric juices, less hydration in their tissues, and changes in subcutaneous fat distribution. They also can have decreased organ capacity for filtration and processing of certain substances, for example in the kidneys and liver. This can affect how medications are digested, stored, and processed out of the body.

Some families of drugs pose a particular risk to this demographic group, which resulted in the Beers list and its guidelines being distributed through national and state health departments to long-term care providers as well as physician and pharmacists who serve elders.

Consumer protection advocate Ralph Nader and others have done extensive research and programs on the issue and have found that most drug abuses, or issues of misuse or overmedication, are not found among youths but in the adult population over 65 years of age. Some of this drug abuse arises as a result of our culture of "I can take a pill for that and be better, right?" and doctors feeling pressured to meet that demand. Some of it arises from the indifference toward elders found in our culture and among some medical professionals, an attitude that it's all downhill and "He is going to die anyway. What am I supposed to do with a 90-year-old?" It is my hope that as we go forward, there will be more progress in the struggle to overcome ageism in our society, patients will be armed with more information and able to guide their own medical care with confidence, and doctors will feel able to make other kinds of suggestions, rather than just prescribing drug options.

OBRA

Another national directive was the passage of the OBRA regulations, which promoted quality of care, resident assessments and care planning and resident rights in long-term care settings, and restricted the use of physical and chemical "neuroleptic" restraints. In that era, both of these care approaches caused a loss of dignity and quality of life for the elder. We were tying elders into their wheelchairs or beds "for their safety." This was an ongoing scary nightmare to a confused elder. The emotional baseline for many individuals in settings using these approaches was fear and anxiety, then when you were approaching them to do a task such as bathing they had no idea what lay ahead.

Defending themselves was a normal and healthy response to the situation. However this was often interpreted by caregivers as acting out and assessed as a need for behavioral drugs. This prompted the OBRA act to tighten prescribing practices regarding frequency and dosages, and creating oversight systems to assure compliance.

TYPES OF MEDICATIONS

The three groups of medications typically used are mood stabilizers (antidepressants, anti-anxiety), anti-psychotics, and anti-convulsive drugs.

Mood Stabilizers

Antidepressants are often prescribed in early stages. Clinicians also want to rule out depression that may be causing a pseudo dementia. That is when a depression causes personality changes, as well as not managing daily life and becoming forgetful and confused. If the antidepressant lifts these symptoms or improves them, this may prove to not be a true dementia or there is a depression overlay that requires treatment to assist maintaining abilities and quality of life. Elders often have faced many losses in life, or have other social, health, or financial concerns that can cause what is called "situational depression." There are also elders who are frightened of seeking help in this area of life, due to the stigma attached to mental illness or they have self-esteem issues around not managing.

Some antidepressant medications can have adverse effects on sexual performance, as some blood pressure medications do, and this may add to the resistance, especially if this area of life remains an active and rewarding part of their primary relationship. Alzheimer's is a depressing thing to face. Individuals aware enough of the changes will need support to handle the situation better. Sometimes antidepressants are part of that support. Counseling with a clinician who understands the importance of expression and doesn't demand retention of the work done from one session to the next, or even within the session, can also be very helpful with discharging the enormous amount of feelings that can arise.

Antidepressants are sometimes also prescribed later in the illness because of increased irritability and not being able to adjust to changing care needs. This can at times give elders a little more resilience handling these situations without using antianxiety meds or antipsychotic. We encourage some families to go this route, especially if there are complicated medical issues or fragilities that warrant attempts to use "little guns" first.

In Middle Stage dementia, it may appear that the elder is not benefiting from the release of endorphins, the brain chemicals that support positive mood, as a result of damage to the brain. We all have difficult times in our lives. If we do not have a problem with depression, we notice that on some mornings we wake up and although nothing has changed in the situation we feel lighter or able to handle things better. It is that piece that seems missing for some elders with dementia. Ongoing problems with brain chemistry and depression are called "clinical depression"; it is different from "situational depression," short-term depression that resolves. There can be a shift from one to the other in an Alzheimer process.

Antipsychotics

Antipsychotics were the first generation of behavioral medications to be developed for psychiatric disorders—a huge, positive step in the treatment of mental illness. But dementia is not a mental illness, even though some phases of the disease can be classified as having psychotic features.

It's true that some individuals may have dual diagnoses: a primary mental illness with secondary developed dementia, and some of these medications have been used with this population. But as was the case with the Beers list, these drugs were tested on younger, healthier individuals, and the dosing approaches are at a much higher level in instances of mental illness.

Many of these early drugs had severe side effects, or "extrapyramidal symptoms," when used on seniors. Symptoms include some or all of the following: increased stiffness, decreased mobility, a stooped posture, shuffling gait, tremors. They can also cause someone to become restless and not be able to stop moving. "Pill rolling" may occur, when the person keeps rubbing their fingers together, as if rolling a pill. Also observed is "cog-wheeling," the staccato-like pattern when the senior is trying to raise their arm or move a leg and rather than a continuous smooth movement, displays little "catches" in the gesture, like the ratcheting of a gear. Another symptom is a mask-like affect, in which the face does not display expression, and drooling and tongue thrusting can also occur.

In the past, practitioners were often using dosage calculations designed to treat schizophrenia in a healthy 35-year-old person and were failing to adjust the dose for a frail, 90-pound, 84-year-old elder with classic delusional thinking related to Alzheimer's disease. Practitioners meant well, but they did not have enough experience yet in dosing for elders with dementia. Nor did they have the benefit of additional research to support their work or any of the new families of drugs we use today. It is only in hindsight that we can see the errors of our ways.

Advanced Alzheimer's disease has many of the features mentioned above as side effects of incorrect dosing—increased stiffness, decreased or increased mobility, and so forth—so in essence, we were progressing individuals through the disease process faster than they would otherwise have done. We were robbing them of a level of participation in their own lives.

Although there may be impairment in the second and third stage of this illness, we still experience individuals able to pursue certain long-standing interests with the right support, able to have fun moments of laughter and positive, loving, and interactive times with families and caregivers. In the past, this was not possible to the degree we see today, due to our understanding of what constituted "best practices" at that time. Hopefully in this field, we will continue to provide more and more humane care as we step into our future each day.

In this light, the approach to use with behavioral meds with individuals with dementia is the least amount of medication possible, dosing at the right times and reviewing periodically to see if a medication should be tapered up or down, depending on the person's current behavioral needs. Side effects should be monitored, and if adverse effects are noted the medication should be reduced, discontinued, or changed.

Anticonvulsants

The use of anticonvulsants is typically indicated in situations where an elder displays unpredictable agitation and a kind of impulsive, volatile, or flaring anger. Individuals who have stroke damage or one of the alcohol-induced dementias can have trouble with this kind of behavior. Other medications may provoke negative reactions, so anticonvulsants may be a better option.

To describe it in lay terms, the chemicals in these drugs treat the areas of the brain that fire inappropriately during a seizure, and quiet brain irritability by helping to turn down the volume on the misfiring, volatile behavior. Side effects can include increased sleepiness, and regular blood work is needed to assess for the risk of toxicity.

GENERAL MEDICATION GUIDANCE

Some folks "go gently into the night," agreeable to assistance, to gentle or friendly correction, to reminders and prompting—these are folks who welcome help and thank caregivers. People like this may never need medications for behaviors, but there was an era when some doctors would order antipsychotics such as Haldol just because the person had an Alzheimer's diagnosis, not because the caregivers were reporting any problems. We saw this especially if there was an admission to hospitals; we see much less of it now.

Thankfully, things have now changed in our understanding of how to work with managing resident behaviors. Much of the focus is first on a good physical assessment, then on the approaches being used, then evaluating the environment to see what is triggering behaviors and what we can do to help create more comfort for the person with memory loss as well as the caregiver. If someone is in pain and this is not being addressed, behaviors may escalate.

Our approach is so important when providing care. Statistically, 50 percent of persons with Alzheimer's become combative at some point in the disease, and 30 percent of them do this when you are doing something they don't want to do. If we adjust our approaches and become more skillful at incorporating their needs and concerns into what we are trying to do this can be reduced. Environments that are understimulating or overstimulating, confusing, or lack safe and natural ways to use energy and express basic aspects of the person's sense of self will cause an increase in difficult behaviors as well.

The last 20 percent of this group may truly have some brain chemistry triggering, causing a fight-or-flight response, or have such poor impulse control they cannot moderate their reactions. When this occurs, it may be necessary to manage the situation with the help of the appropriate medications in order to help with safety and quality of life. The goal is never to overmedicate or sedate someone so that their normal level of functioning lessens. But it may take some trial and error, with periodic adjustments, to find a supportive medication approach for behavioral needs.

Some families may need to get referrals for different professionals to handle specific medications. In some cases, a primary care physician may ask for a consult with a specialist in the area of gerontology or with a psychiatrist or neurologist. Some Health Maintenance Organizations (HMOs) will suggest a psychiatric nurse or nurse practitioner be brought in. It may also be possible to draw on the expertise of a local mental health team supported by county or state funding services, which includes geriatric psychologists or psychiatrists, social workers, and/or nurses.

Make sure that these practitioners take as much time as you need to answer your questions about the medications and teach you what your options are and how to understand the difference between a short-acting medication and a long-acting medication. For example, if the elder is displaying heightened anxiety or agitation associated with specific tasks that occur at specific times, a short-acting medication may be appropriate, such as the anti-anxiety medications ativan or lorazapam.

Note: Anti-anxiety medications can cause some frail elders to fall, and many physicians may not use them for that reason. However if you have a loved one with great balance, good vitality, and you are only having trouble three times a week on shower day this may be a good option. Using a low dose, 30 minutes before suggesting or attempting this task, can reduce resistance and cause the person to be calm enough to get the bath done. The drug usually clears from the body's blood and nervous system within one to two hours, and the person can return to their baseline or normal behavior.

Some individuals have problems with dental appointments or lab work, so the use of this medication is infrequent; others may have daily escalations in behaviors as a result of what's known as "sundowning," becoming agitated as night falls. In this case, the caregiver may need to estimate the peak of this daily agitation and aim to give the med each afternoon in advance of this escalation.

When someone's behavior is unpredictable, and the caregiver is unable to find triggering causes they can adjust, a drug that stays in the body for longer periods and over time helps the person remain calmer and less agitated may be needed. These medications are considered long-acting drugs.

QUESTION YOUR DOCTOR
When you are discussing these medications with your specialist, ask the following questions:
- Which drugs, and at what dosages, will be needed in order to affect blood levels, and how long will it take to see behavioral differences?
- How long do the medications remain in the system once they have been discontinued? (Some drugs take up to six weeks to clear out of the body after they are stopped.)
- What are the positive and negative effects of the drugs?

- Will they initially make someone more drowsy or dizzy, and how long will it take for this effect to wear off and for the person to become used to the medication? (This is typically about three days.)
- What would be really bad side effects that mean the person should stop taking the medication right away, and the best approach to contact the professional?
- Is there a rotation of responders in the practice to answer after-hours calls? What is their schedule? If after-hours responders are not available during this initial adjustment, would it be okay to contact the doctor directly?
- What is the level of cooperation, understanding, and ability of the person who takes calls on weekends or at night?
- Which medications have a withdrawal problem?
- What is the doctor's suggestion for a tapering dosage reduction, if for some reason the doctor is going to be unavailable, e.g., on vacation or maternity leave? (Sometimes persons on call do not want to get involved in changing or adjusting medications if they have not worked with your loved one, or don't have the skill set. They will therefore be unable or unwilling to discuss this with you if the need arises.)

Because the person with dementia is on a path of progression, things will continue to change. Sometimes these changes signal less need for medications. The person with memory loss has passed through a phase of heightened sensitivity, and the things that caused them to respond with anxiety or agitation are no longer producing that behavior. There may be a period later when the need arises again for behavioral medications, but we should be looking for ways to reduce medications whenever possible.

At some point, use of medications may produce what is called a "paradoxical effect." This is when the medication causes the opposite response to what was intended. The goal in giving the medication may have been to calm someone down, but now after taking it, they are more agitated. Discuss this with the prescribing clinician as soon as you note this.

ASK FOR HELP

Over many years of working with physicians and specialists in this field, I have run into practitioners who are not familiar with the progression of Alzheimer's disease, and do not particularly understand or have compassion for the dementia process. They tend to be somewhat rigid in the medications they prescribe and are not great listeners when it comes to feedback from the caregivers. They may also change too many medications at once, or change them too quickly, not allowing results to guide the next adjustment. They may go right to the "big guns" when "lighter weight" medications, i.e., those with less side effects, may be sufficient. On the other hand, they may go the other way and not want to order anything, leaving the caregiver with no options for an increasingly difficult or unsafe situation.

Do not be afraid to get a second opinion. Ask for dementia-friendly doctor referrals from your local Alzheimer's association, or support group, or other family members you may know who have traveled or are traveling this same path. Call local home care or hospice agencies, or nursing care centers and ask to speak with an experienced nurse in their team who works with memory care patients and their families. See if they have some recommendations for who is good to work with in your community. This is very important to the care of your loved one and to you. It will alleviate some of the angst of caregiving if you feel trusting and confident in the specialist who is assisting you.

Bibliography

Bell, Virginia, and David Troxel. *The Best Friends™ Approach to Alzheimer's Care.* Baltimore, MD: Health Professions Press, 1997.

Bell, Virginia, and David Troxel. *A Dignified Life: The Best Friends™ Approach to Alzheimer's Care: A Guide for Family Caregivers.* Revised expanded edition. Deerfield Beach, FL: HCI Books, 2012.

Bell, Virginia, David Troxel, Tonya Cox, and Robin Hamon. *The Best Friends™ Book of Alzheimer's Activities:147 Fun, Easy, and Enriching Activities.* Vol. 1. Baltimore, MD: Health Professions Press, 2009.

Bianco, Margery Williams, and Allen Atkinson. *The Velveteen Rabbit.* New York, NY: Alfred A. Knopf, 1983.

Brennan, Barbara Ann. *Hands of Light: A Guide to Healing Through the Human Energy Field: A New Paradigm for the Human Being in Health, Relationship, and Disease.* Toronto, Canada: Bantam Books, 1988.

Brokaw, Tom. *The Greatest Generation.* New York, NY: Random House, 1998.

Chishti, N.D., Hakim G. M. *The Traditional Healer's Handbook: A Classic Guide to the Medicine of Avicenna.* Rochester, VT: Healing Arts Press, 1991.

_____. *The Book of Sufi Healing.* Revised edition. Rochester, VT: Inner Traditions/Bear and Company, 1985.

Cohen, Ken. *Honoring the Medicine: The Essential Guide to Native American Healing.* New York, NY: Ballantine Books, 2003. (Direct quotes from text with permission of the author.)

Descartes, Renee, and John Veitch. *Selections from the Principles of Philosophy.* Ottawa, Canada: eBooksLib.com, 2011.

Diamond, Jared. *The World Until Yesterday: What We Can Learn from Traditional Societies.* New York, NY: Viking Penguin Group, 2012.

Dossey, Larry. *Prayer is Good Medicine: How to Reap the Healing Benefits of Prayer.* San Francisco, CA: HarperSanFrancisco, 1996.

_____. *Healing Beyond the Body: Medicine and the Infinite Reach of the Mind.* Boston, MA: Shambhala, 2001.

Dychtwald, Ken, and Joe Flower. *Age Wave: The Challenges and Opportunities of an Aging America.* Los Angeles, CA: J.P. Tarcher, 1989.

Feil, Naomi, and Vicki de Rubin. *The Validation Breakthrough: Simple Techniques for Communicating with People with Alzheimer's and Other Dementias.* 3rd ed. Baltimore, MD: Health Professions Press, 2012.

Kazantzakis, Nikos. *God's Pauper: St. Francis of Assisi: A Novel.* Oxford, UK: Cassirer, 1975.

Mace, Nancy L., and Peter V. Rabins. *The 36-Hour Day: A Family Guide to Caring for People with Alzheimer's Disease, Other Dementias, and Memory Loss in Later Life.* 4th ed. Baltimore, MD: Johns Hopkins University Press, 2006.

Maslow, Abraham. *Motivation and Personality.* New York. NY: Harper 1954.

Nightingale, Florence. *Notes on Nursing: What It Is, and What It Is Not.* Commemorative ed. Philadelphia, PA: Lippincott, 1992.

Sartre, Jean. *Being and Nothingness: An Essay on Phenomenological Ontology.* New York, NY: Philosophical Library, 1956.

Snowdon, David. *Aging with Grace: What the Nun Study Teaches Us About Leading Longer, Healthier, and More Meaningful Lives.* New York, NY: Bantam Books, 2001.

Steiner, Rudolf, and Paul Marshall Allen. *Truth and Knowledge: Introduction to Philosophy of Spiritual Activity.* 2nd ed. Blauvelt, NY: Steinerbooks, 1981.

Thomas, William H. *Life Worth Living: How Someone You Love Can Still Enjoy Life in a Nursing Home: The Eden Alternative in Action.* Acton, MA: VanderWyk & Burnham, 1996.

Williams, Margery. Original illustrations by William Nicholson. *The Velveteen Rabbit: Or How Toys Become Real.* Deerfield Beach, FL: HCI Books. First published by Heinneman in 1922. New edition 2005.

Further Information

Alzheimer's Association. www.alz.org

Alzheimer's Disease International. http://www.alz.co.uk

American Horticultural Therapy Association. http://ahta.org

American Massage Therapy Association. http://www.amtamassage.org/index.html

American Stroke Association. www.strokeassociation.org

Anthroposophical Medicine. http://www.paam.net/anthroposophical-medicine

Association for Frontotemporal Degeneration RSS. http://www.theaftd.org

Creutzfeldt-Jakob Disease Foundation. http://www.cjdfoundation.org

Parkinson's Disease Foundation (PDF). http://www.pdf.org

Lewy Body Dementia Association. http://www.lbda.org

Lupus Foundation of America. http://www.lupus.org

American Cancer Society. http://www.cancer.org

American Diabetes Association. http://www.diabetes.org

American Heart Association. www.heart.org

American Psychiatric Association. http://www.psych.org

Camphill Communities of North America. http://www.camphill.org

Camphill Worldwide. http://camphill.net

Equestrian Therapy. http://www.equestriantherapy.com

Live Oak Institute. http://www.liveoakinstitute.org

Meals On Wheels Association of America. https://www.mowaa.org

National Association for Holistic Aromatherapy. https://www.naha.org

Pioneer Network. http://www.pioneernetwork.net

Planetree. http://planetree.org

Good Old Days Magazine. http://www.goodolddaysmagazine.com/